YOGA
OF LIGHT

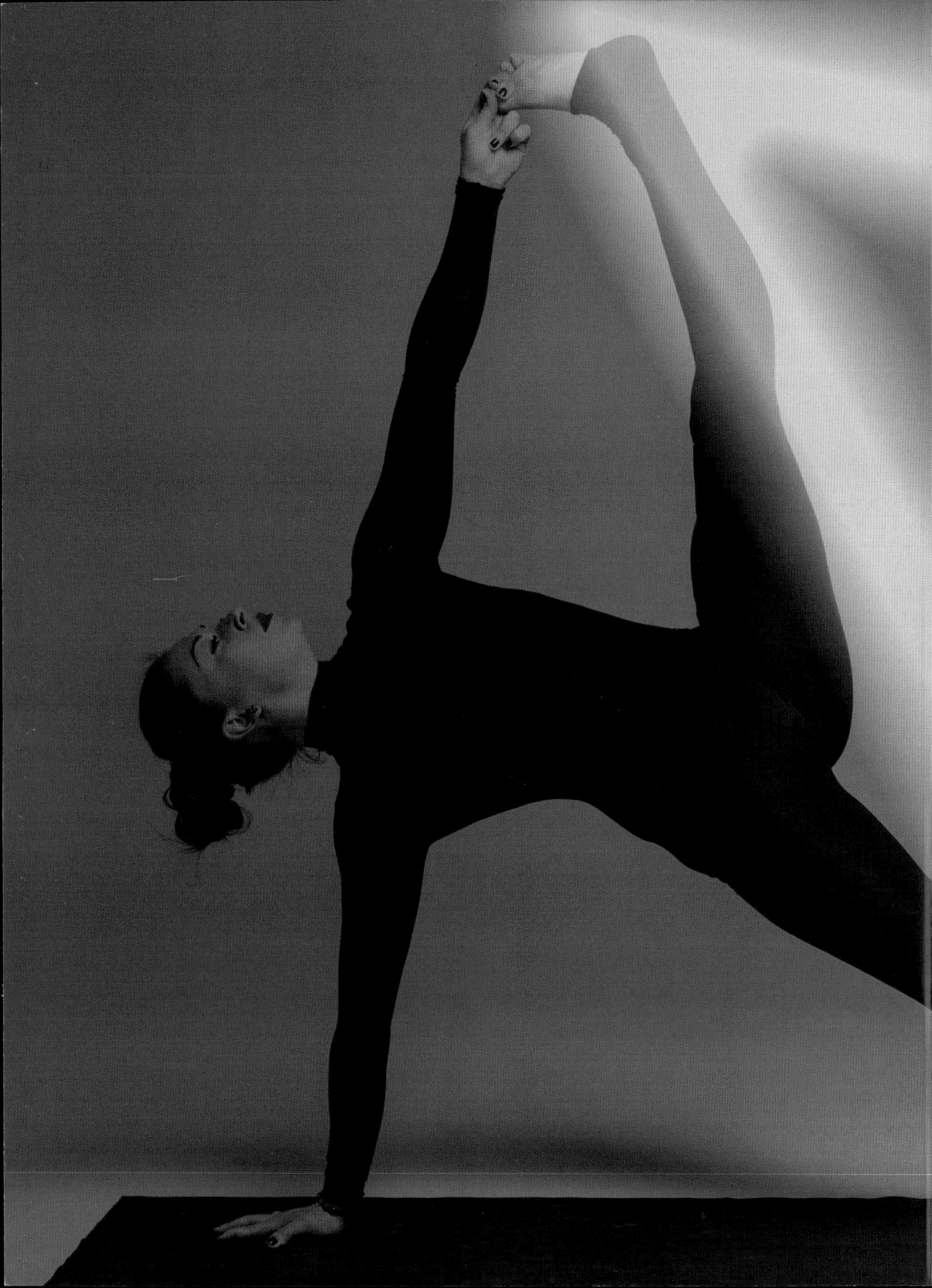

PAULINE WILLS

YOGA
OF LIGHT

AWAKEN
CHAKRA ENERGIES
THROUGH THE
TRIANGLES OF LIGHT

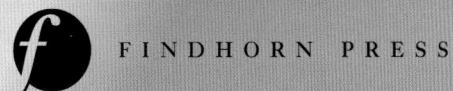
FINDHORN PRESS

Findhorn Press
One Park Street
Rochester, Vermont 05767
www.findhornpress.com

Findhorn Press is a division of Inner Traditions International

Text copyright © Pauline Wills 2019
Original edition copyright © Eddison Books Limited 2019
www.eddisonbooks.com

This edition published by Findhorn Press in 2019
by arrangement with Eddison Books Limited.

Disclaimer
The information in this book is given in good faith and is neither intended to
diagnose any physical or mental condition nor to serve as a substitute for informed
medical advice or care. Please contact your health professional for medical advice
and treatment. Neither author nor publisher can be held liable by any person for
any loss or damage whatsoever which may arise from the use of this book or any
of the information therein.

Cataloging-in-Publication data for this title is available from the Library of Congress

ISBN 978-1-62055-944-4 (print)
ISBN 978-1-62055-945-1 (ebook)

1 3 5 7 9 10 8 6 4 2

Printed in Serbia

CONTENTS

INTRODUCTION 6

CHAPTER 1   **WHAT IS YOGA? 8**

CHAPTER 2   **THE WEB OF LIGHT 23**

CHAPTER 3   **THE CHAKRAS 31**

CHAPTER 4   **PRANAYAMA 55**

CHAPTER 5   **WORKING WITH THE CHAKRAS 69**

CHAPTER 6   **THE TRIANGLES OF LIGHT 89**

INDEX 158

ACKNOWLEDGEMENTS 160

INTRODUCTION

Yoga is one of the earliest-known belief systems, combining spiritual awareness with physical discipline. It's believed that most paths or religions have absorbed at least some of its teachings. Yoga's principles are based on the eight steps of yoga laid down by the Eastern sage Patanjali. These encompass restraints and observances, posture, breathing, concentration, contemplation and meditation. In the West, unfortunately, yoga tends to be looked on solely as a keep-fit routine. The asanas, or postures, do, indeed, encourage physical fitness, but this is far from yoga's true essence.

When practising an asana, the position of the body must be precise, in order for the posture to work with the body's energy centres, or chakras. The emphasis isn't on how many times a posture is formed but on how long that posture is held, while maintaining the correct breathing, sustained concentration on the posture and contemplation of the relevant chakra or chakras.

Through working and teaching in this way for the past twenty-five years, I began first to feel lines of energy linking the chakras and then to 'see' this energy as triangles of light. When this first occurred, I had no idea what was happening or what these triangles indicated. It was only through meditating on what I was experiencing, and researching little-known works on yoga philosophy, that I began to learn that these triangles form as we evolve spiritually and our chakras start to clear and open. The journey has been exciting. But at times it has also been challenging, both physically, as the chakras cleansed themselves of old debris accumulated over many lifetimes, and in the changes that this cleansing brought about on all levels of being.

One of the main chakras involved in the creation of these triangles of light is the alta major, situated where the cervical spine enters the skull. This chakra is sometimes called 'The Mouth of God', because it's here that pranic, or life force, energy is fed into the body to energize and maintain it. Enlightened beings reputed to have lived for years without taking food or water are believed to have sustained the physical body with the energy that enters the body through the alta major chakra. Initially, when these triangles of light start to form, they're felt either as heat or as a tingling sensation. It's only constant practice, combined with meditation, that enables us to 'see' them with our inner sight. We are, I believe, beings of light, and it's these triangles that amplify the light of our true being.

More and more people now believe that the present period in Earth's history is a time when our planet and all things living upon it are being challenged to make a quantum leap out of our three-dimensional world into a fourth and fifth dimension. For this to occur, old structures have to be broken down to create space for a new way of living and being. I believe that the triangles of light formed within our bodies are part of that transformation process – a process that heightens the frequency to which each of us resonates and, in so doing, aids and prepares us for that quantum leap.

For those who wish to work with the triangles of light, you must face some challenges and be happy to make changes in your life. If you're prepared to do this, these triangles can build up your own inner light and eventually lead you to a state of enlightenment.

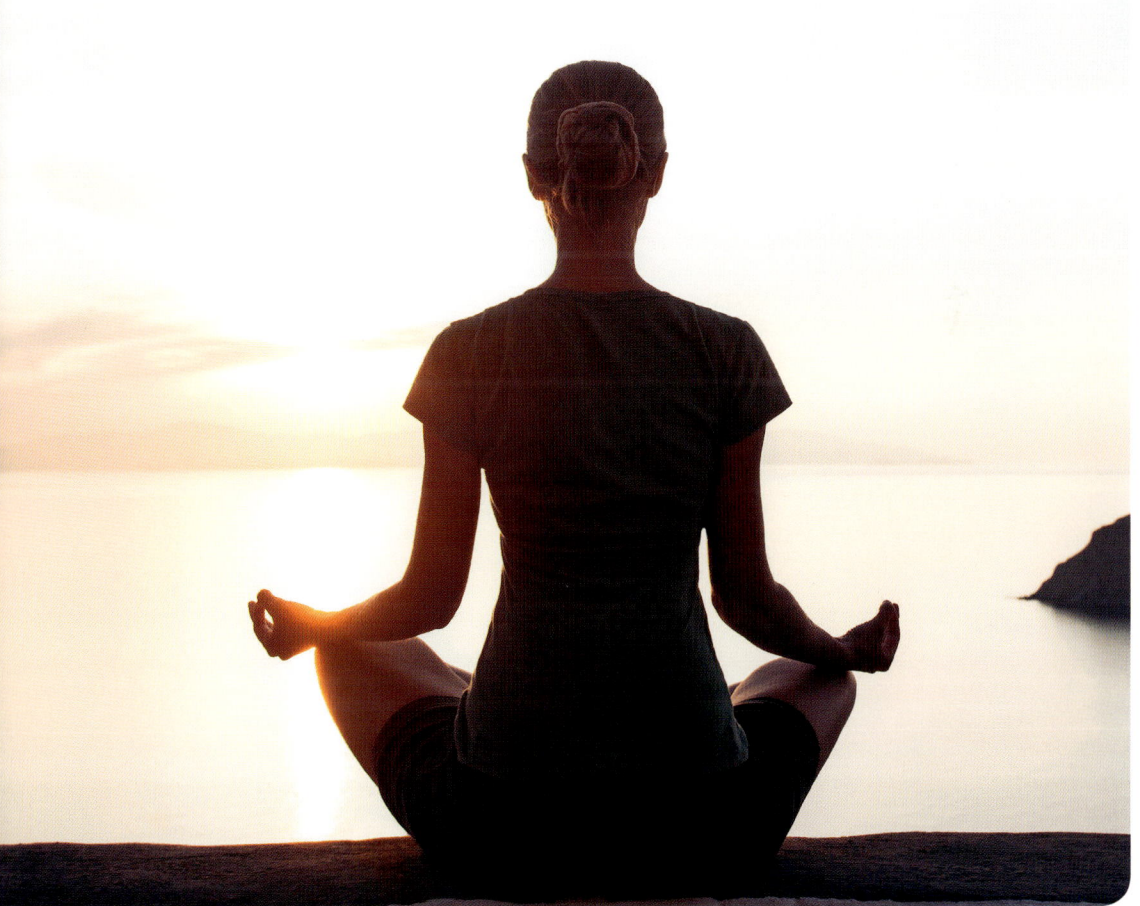

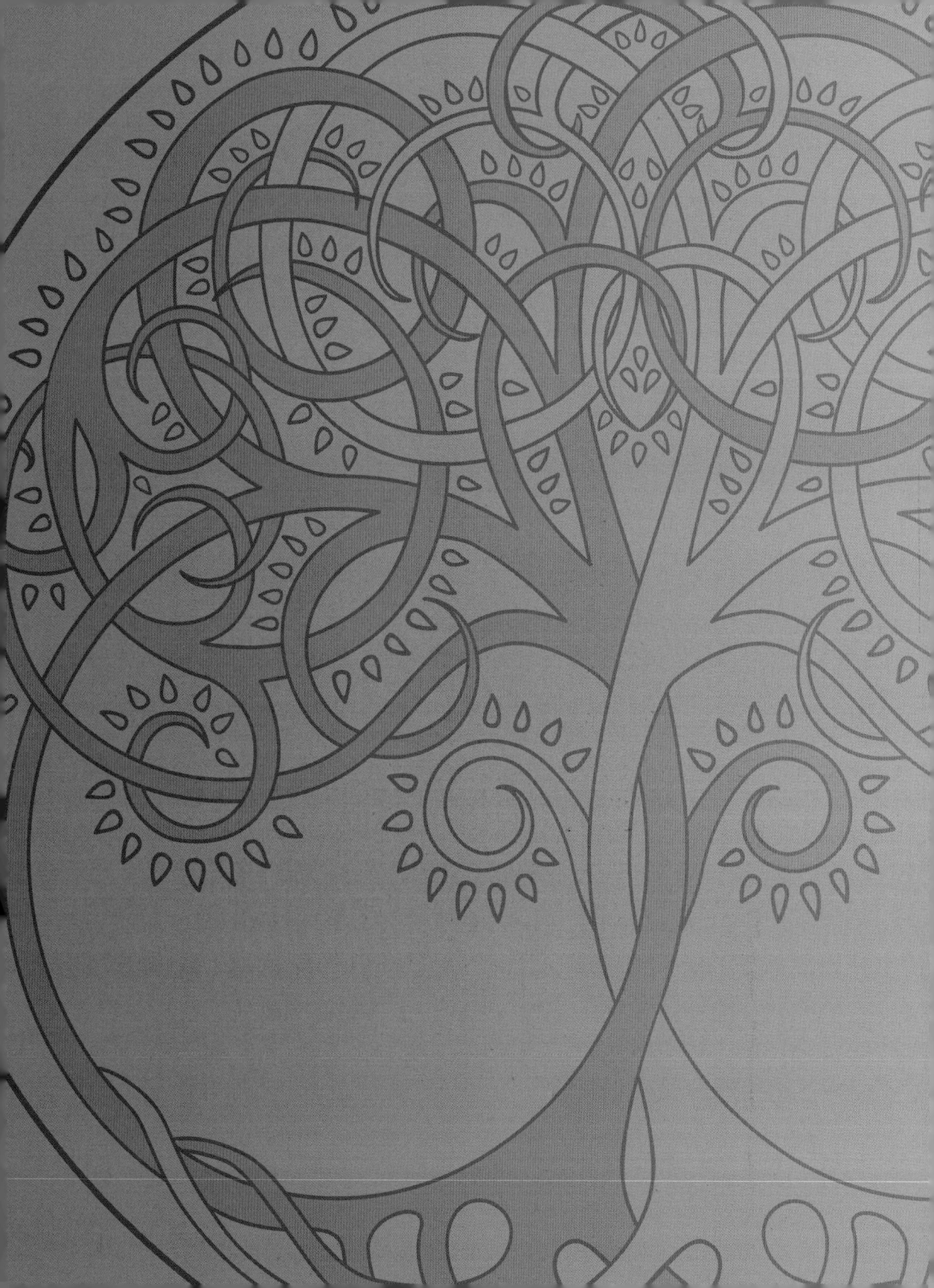

1

WHAT IS YOGA?

YOGA IS A DISCIPLINE – A WAY OF LIFE THAT
AIMS TO HELP US REALIZE OUR TRUE SELF: THAT
ETERNAL ELEMENT OF US THAT IS PART OF THE
CREATOR OF THE UNIVERSE, THE SUPREME
REALITY THAT HAS NO BEGINNING AND NO END;
THE INEXTINGUISHABLE ESSENCE THAT'S PRESENT
IN ALL LIFE. YOGA PREACHES NO DOGMA, BUT
WILL ENHANCE ANY RELIGION OR PATH THAT
A PERSON CHOOSES TO FOLLOW.

THE STORY AND ESSENCE OF YOGA

The word 'yoga' derives from the Sanskrit *yug*, meaning 'to unite', and in the practice of yoga we unite body, mind and spirit into wholeness, in order to reach samadhi, a state of deep contemplation, leading to higher understanding and consciousness. This is why one of the questions that yoga students are invited to ask themselves is 'Who am I?' – or, as the twentieth-century spiritualist Paul Brunton preferred to say in his book *The Hidden Teaching Beyond Yoga*, 'What am I?'

Yoga is ancient. Some of its earliest traces were uncovered in the 1920s during excavations led by archeologist Sir John Marshall at Mohenjo-daro in the Indus Valley, including sculptures of human figures and two glazed pottery seals more than 4,000 years old. The first of these faience seals depicted a man seated in the lotus posture, flanked by two worshippers with raised and folded hands. The second seal showed a man in the lotus posture, seated on a pedestal and surrounded by an elephant, a lion, a buffalo, a rhinoceros and a pair of deer. One of the excavated sculptures was of a man meditating in full lotus posture; another sculpture, depicting only the upper part of the body, was of a bearded, long-haired figure with his eyes closed in meditation and a cloth thrown across one shoulder. Similar figures have been found in the ancient city of Harappa, also in the Indus Valley, dated to the third millennium BCE.

Yoga, like a tree, has many branches, all ultimately supporting each other to create wholeness. The earliest branch of the tree, representing the first yogic path, is jnana yoga, the yoga of wisdom and knowledge. Its first literary exposition appears in the *Upanishads*, a collection of texts from the first century BCE that's still used and valued today. Said to have been composed through meditation, the writings of the *Upanishads* iterate the important role that meditation plays in equipping the practitioner for the great intuitive revelation that the texts reveal. However, beautiful though the *Upanishads* are, many feel they lack the warmth and comfort found in the later ancient Indian classics the *Bhagavad-Gita* and the great sage Patanjali's *Yoga Sutras*.

No one is sure precisely when Patanjali lived, although some scholars have dated his existence to around 300 BCE. All the main practices of yoga are included in Patanjali's sutras – pithy sayings that were initially passed by word of mouth from master to student, who was then expected to meditate upon their meaning. Encompassed within the sutras are the eight limbs of yoga on which its practice is based. In his sutras, Patanjali explains that following the eight steps of yoga removes impurities from the body and mind in preparation for experiencing the light of the true self. These eight yogic steps are the yamas, the niyamas, the asanas, pranayama, pratyahara, dharana, dhyana and samadhi.

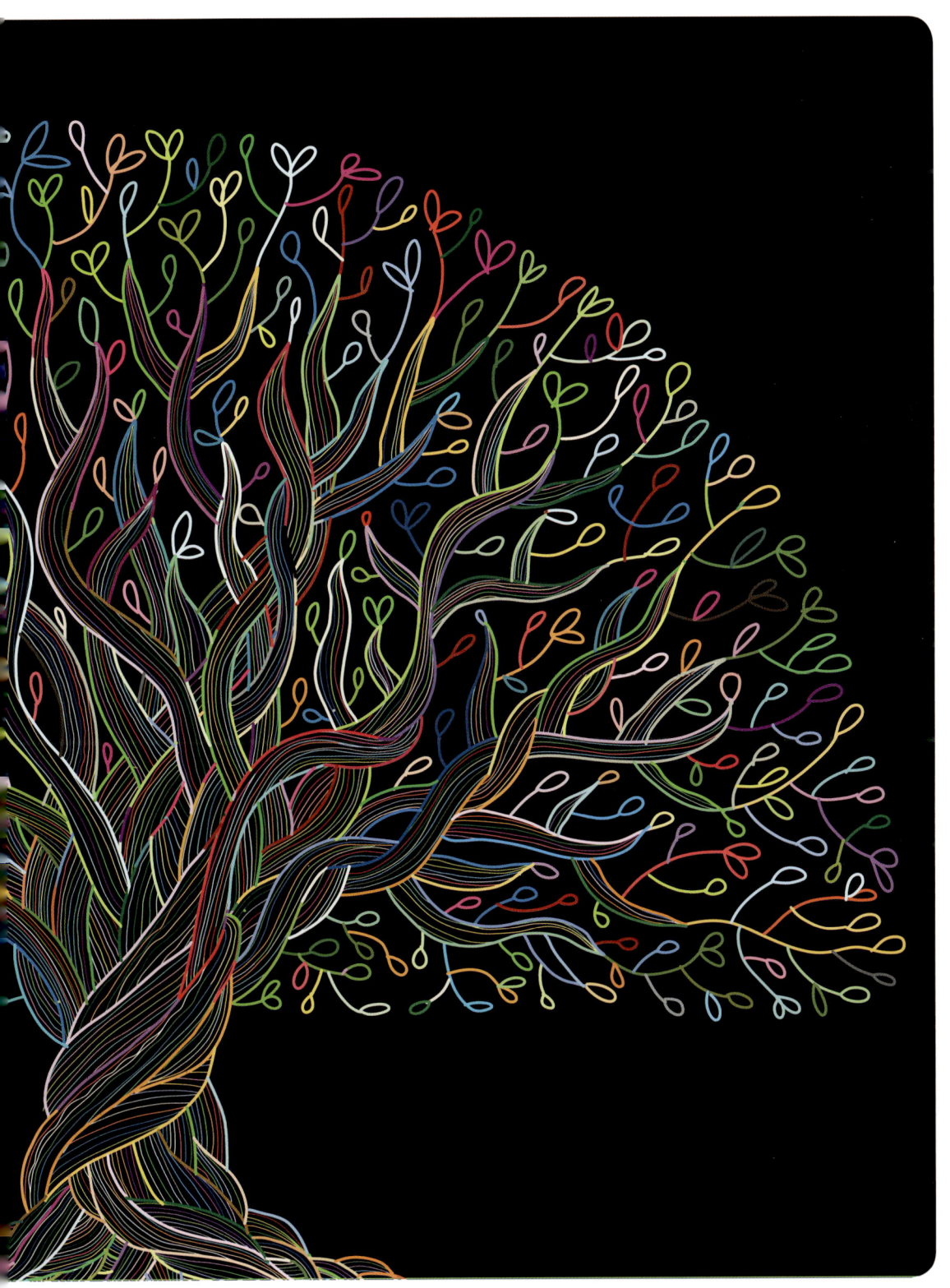

THE EIGHT STEPS OF YOGA

YAMAS
The first step – the five yamas, or ethical disciplines

AHIMSA (non-violence)
Yogis believe that all living creatures contain the essence of God within them, making their earthly form sacred. If this is so, a bond is created that links us to each other. Therefore, if we harm or injure others, we're also harming ourselves. Frequently, I hear students protest that they're in no way physically violent. This may be true – but we can be just as violent with our thoughts. Violence springs from negative thoughts or feelings, such as hatred, jealousy, fear and anger. If we have such feelings, then we're devoid of love. It's only through love of ourselves and others that we can truly start to practise ahimsa.

SATYA (truthfulness)
Truth begins with being truthful to ourselves, acknowledging both our talents and our faults. Only when we acknowledge our faults can we work to overcome them; and once we look truthfully at ourselves, it's much easier to look truthfully at others. When we follow the path of yoga, we should practise truthfulness not only in our thoughts but also in our actions and speech. Untruthfulness in speech includes abuse, obscenity and telling lies, but also the ridiculing of what others hold to be sacred. Untruthfulness in action lies in doing things that we know to be wrong for us.

ASTEYA (non-stealing)
The asteya yama applies to many of the things that we do in our everyday life. If we take from others things that don't belong to us, we're not only stealing – we're also not practising ahimsa. If we tell untruths about other people, we're not only failing to practise truthfulness – we're also stealing their reputation by forging false evidence.

BRAMACHARYA (chastity)
The literal translation of bramacharya is 'a life of celibacy' – but this doesn't mean that a practising yogi must refrain from sex (unless they want to). The Indian yogi Paramahansa Yogananda says in his book *Man's Eternal Quest* that sexual intercourse is the highest expression of love within the married state or between committed partners. But he also explains that the sexual act shouldn't take place merely for self-gratification. In his book *Sexual Force or the Winged Dragon*, the Bulgarian philosopher

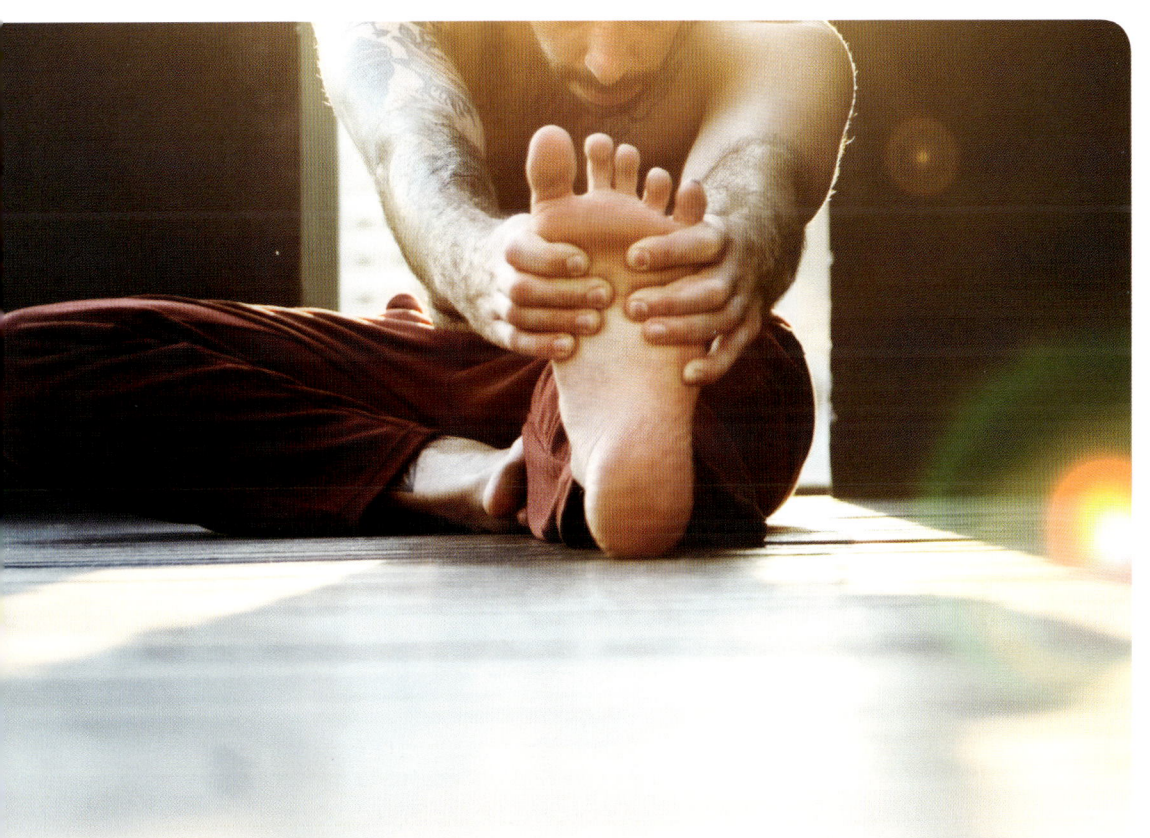

and mystic Omraam Mikhaël Aïvanhov states that instead of using our sexual energy for pleasure, we should transmute it into our higher energy centres to help us reach the state of enlightenment. Transmuting sexual energy is part of the practice of tantric yoga, and its purpose is to raise the latent energy, or kundalini, that resides in the base chakra. It's important, however, to realize that tantric yoga can be dangerous if it isn't taught by a teacher far advanced in the practice.

APARIGRAHA (non-acquisitiveness)

Simply put, aparigraha means that we shouldn't hoard or collect things that we don't need. Amassing earthly goods can be addictive, and the more we amass, the more we want. Earthly goods only give us transient pleasure. The gratification provided by our latest acquisition soon vanishes, leaving us craving for a new and seemingly brighter object. Remember that we came into the world with nothing, and we're going to leave with nothing – so why collect possessions that we don't really need? I believe that if we're following a spiritual path and trying to help others in whatever way we can, we'll be given what we need when we need it. Patanjali says in his sutras that 'one who has rid himself of "I" and "mine"' is able to see themselves in their proper perspective.

NIYAMAS
The second step – the five niyamas, or rules of conduct

SAUCHA (cleanliness)

The cleanliness of our physical body is essential for our well-being. We all know how important it is to bathe regularly and to wear clean clothes, but saucha also braces internal cleanliness. Practising the asanas or postures tones our muscles and removes toxins and impurities; the breathing exercises oxygenate our blood and calm our nerves. Equally important is diet. Ideally, food should be eaten to strengthen the body and provide it with the vitamins and minerals it needs to function to its full potential. This requires a balanced, wholesome diet, free from processed, devitalized food. When we become sensitive to our body's needs, we instinctively know what to eat at any given time. Unfortunately, the pace and pressures of modern life have got many of us into the habit of basing our diet mainly on fast food and a quick appeal to the taste buds. It's easy, therefore, to forget that we are what we eat.

Another important aspect of saucha is cleansing the mind of negative emotions, such as hatred, envy, anger, delusion and pride. Like attracts like, and if we send out negative, unclean thoughts we'll attract the same kind of thoughts back to ourselves. We need also to remember that our thoughts influence our body in the same way that our body affects our mind.

SANTOSA (contentment)

Contentment and tranquillity are states of mind. To reach true contentment, we have to free ourselves from desire, learn to live in the present and trust that if we're seeking a union with that ultimate reality, whatever name we want to give it, we'll receive what we need when we need it. Amassing possessions can lead to a lack of contentment. The more we own, the more we have to worry about. The true contentment of santosa is found in a simple, uncluttered life.

TAPAS (austerity and spritual practice)

The name of this niyama comes from the Sanskrit verb *tap*, meaning to burn or consume by heat. In a yogic context, it means a burning effort to achieve the final step of yoga – samadhi or God consciousness – by committing to the fire of purification our desires and negativity, and anything else that stands in our way. B.K.S. Iyengar, originator of Iyengar yoga, says in his book *Light on Yoga* that life without tapas is like a heart without love.

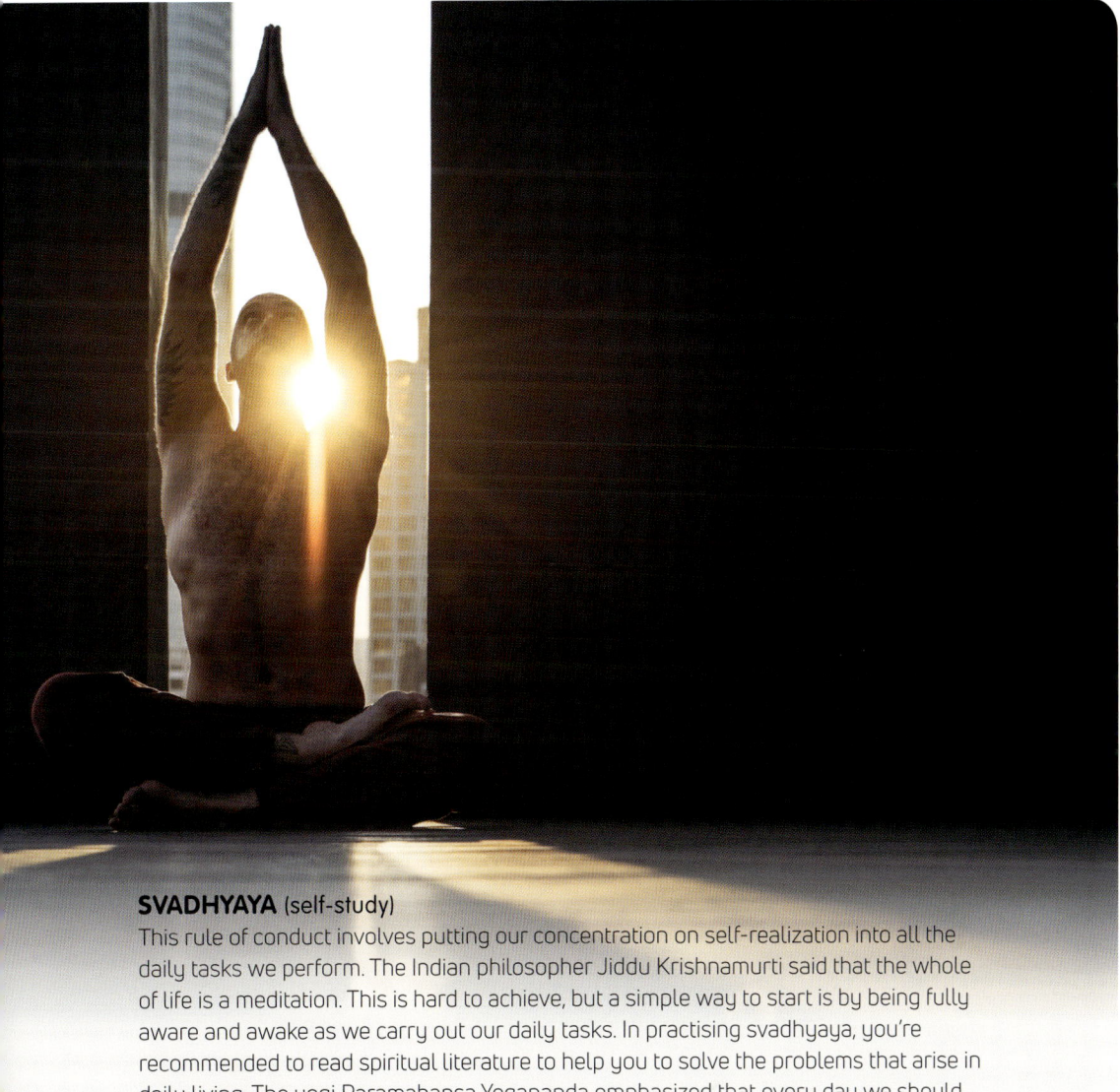

SVADHYAYA (self-study)

This rule of conduct involves putting our concentration on self-realization into all the daily tasks we perform. The Indian philosopher Jiddu Krishnamurti said that the whole of life is a meditation. This is hard to achieve, but a simple way to start is by being fully aware and awake as we carry out our daily tasks. In practising svadhyaya, you're recommended to read spiritual literature to help you to solve the problems that arise in daily living. The yogi Paramahansa Yogananda emphasized that every day we should begin and end with God, by coming into the deity's presence through meditation.

ISVARA PRANIDHANA (attentiveness to God)

Here we accept all our experiences as coming from God. These experiences are the challenges that prepare us to open to the God light that resides within each of us. We should see God in everything we do, and include that divine being in all our thoughts. By centring our mind on God, the thoughts that boost our ego are banished.

ASANAS
The third step – the postures of yoga

Asana, from the Sanskrit word for 'seat', means to hold the body firmly in a particular position, while focusing on the energy centre, or centres, with which the posture works. Practising asanas brings suppleness to the body, strengthens and detoxifies the muscles, frees the body from disease, steadies the mind, clears the chakras of accumulated debris and brings lightness to your being. An asana is perfected when effort ceases and you reach a state of bliss. Through dedicated practice of the asanas, together with practice of the other yoga steps, the chakras start to link with each other, creating triangles of light. Initially, you visualize these triangles while holding the posture, then, with continued practice, you start to feel the triangles and, finally, you're able to see them with your inner vision. I believe that the triangles play an important part in our initiation into the higher levels of consciousness. Also, they increase the light energy within us and initiate us into what we truly are – beings of light. The key asanas are shown in Chapter 6.

PRANAYAMA
The fourth step – breath control

Prana is the life force and *yama* means the expansion of its length, breadth and volume. There are many pranayama exercises, and, when performed correctly, they are said to eradicate all disease from the body, to regulate the pulse, bring radiance to the complexion, quieten the mind and increase the intake of oxygen. There are three important aspects to breath control: exhalation (*recaka*), inhalation (*puranas*) and retention (*kumbhaka*). These are explained in greater detail in Chapter 4.

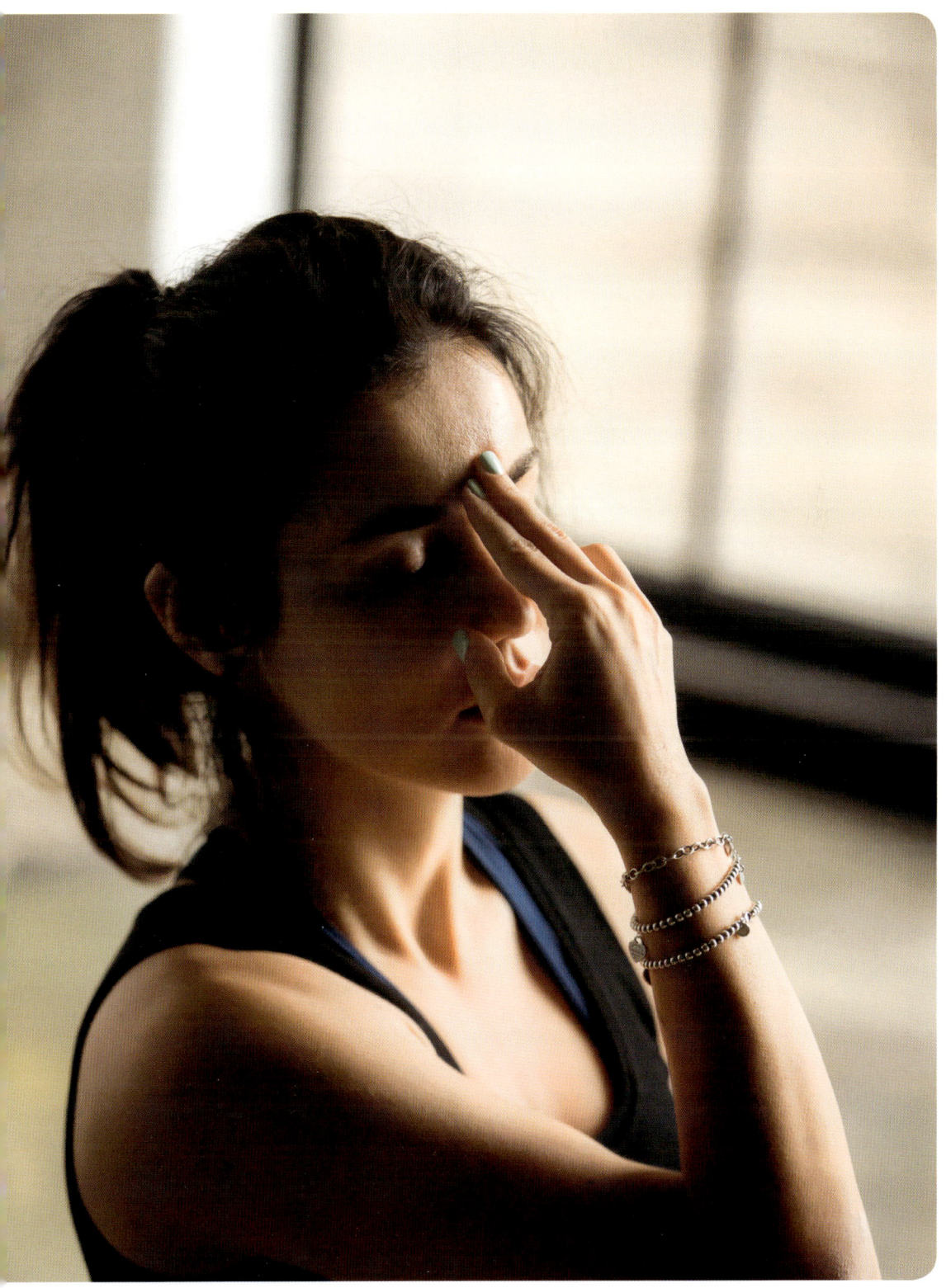

PRATYAHARA
The fifth step – control of the senses

This step involves withdrawing the mind from the sense organs to tune into our true self without distraction from the external world. The yogi Paramahansa Yogananda taught his disciples to place a thumb in each ear and the remaining fingers over the eyes when starting to practise pratyahara. Closing and covering the eyes prevents us from seeing external objects; closing our ears shuts out external noise.

DHARANA
The sixth step – concentration

For most of us, the mind is our master, constantly wandering through a variety of subjects and over events that have taken place or are about to do so. Therefore, when we initially attempt to reverse roles and become the master of our mind, our mind rebels. My yoga master used to say that we needed a sense of humour to practise this particular system, because if we allowed it to make us frustrated, our concentration would worsen. He always jokingly advised that we treat our mind like a naughty child. Each time it wandered away from the object of concentration, we had to gently bring it back. A technique taught by the spiritual teacher Ekhart Tolle is to spend several minutes each day practising living in the present – in the now. He says that if we practise for 30 seconds twice a day, that's good. If we practise for 1 minute twice a day, that's very good, and if we practise for longer, that's excellent. This is a very good exercise to try. It's mastery of dharana that leads us gently into the seventh step of yoga – dhyana.

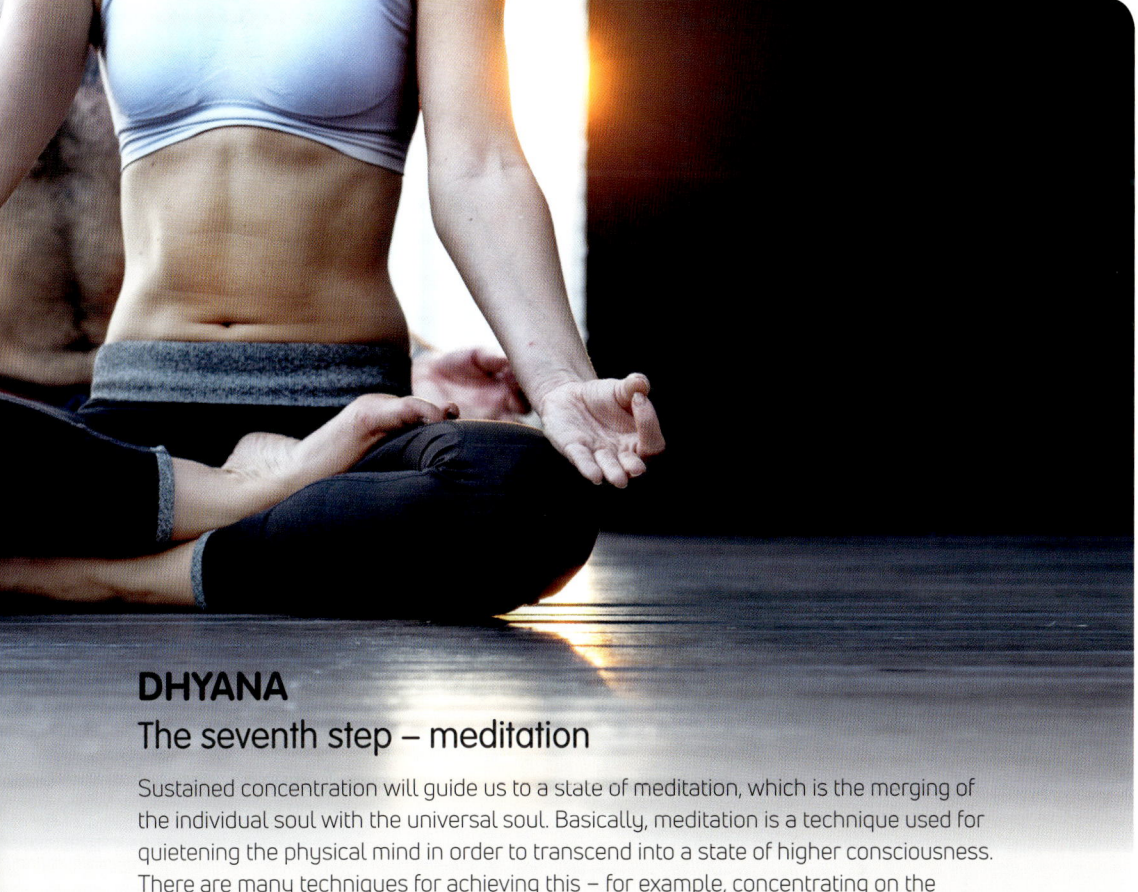

DHYANA
The seventh step – meditation

Sustained concentration will guide us to a state of meditation, which is the merging of the individual soul with the universal soul. Basically, meditation is a technique used for quietening the physical mind in order to transcend into a state of higher consciousness. There are many techniques for achieving this – for example, concentrating on the breath – a technique recommended by many yogic masters because the breath is always with us; working with a sound (mantra), or a diagram or pattern (mandala); or using visualization. Some of these techniques are explained in Chapter 3.

SAMADHI
The eighth step – self-realization

Many of the yoga masters describe this as a state of pure bliss, free from all the trappings of the world and the physical body. It's the merging of our true self with the supreme. The Christ described this when he said, 'I and my Father are one'. This state can take many lifetimes to achieve, but once attained there's no longer any need to reincarnate into this world unless we want to help others to come to the state of self-realization.

WORKING WITH THE STEPS

Many of the eight steps can be incorporated into the practice of just one. For example, before practising asanas, which ideally should be done first thing in the morning, we should take a shower. We can incorporate the correct breathing that goes with the posture, and withdraw our senses from the external world to fully concentrate on what we're doing. If we strain a muscle through lack of concentration, then we haven't practised ahimsa. We can make sure that each part of the body maintains the correct position throughout the length of time we're holding the posture; the longer a posture is held, the greater the effect it has on the energy centres or chakras it's working with, and the greater the energy the posture generates.

As mentioned earlier, yoga is a discipline, a way of life. It's only through practice that you'll begin to reap its benefits. In the *Bhagavad-Gita* it says:

Yoga is a harmony. Not for him who eats too much or for him who eats too little; not for him who sleeps too little; nor for him who sleeps too much. A harmony in eating and resting, in sleeping and keeping awake: a perfection in whatever one does. This is the yoga that gives peace from all pain. And the greatest of all yogis is he who with all his soul has faith, and he who with all his soul loves Me.

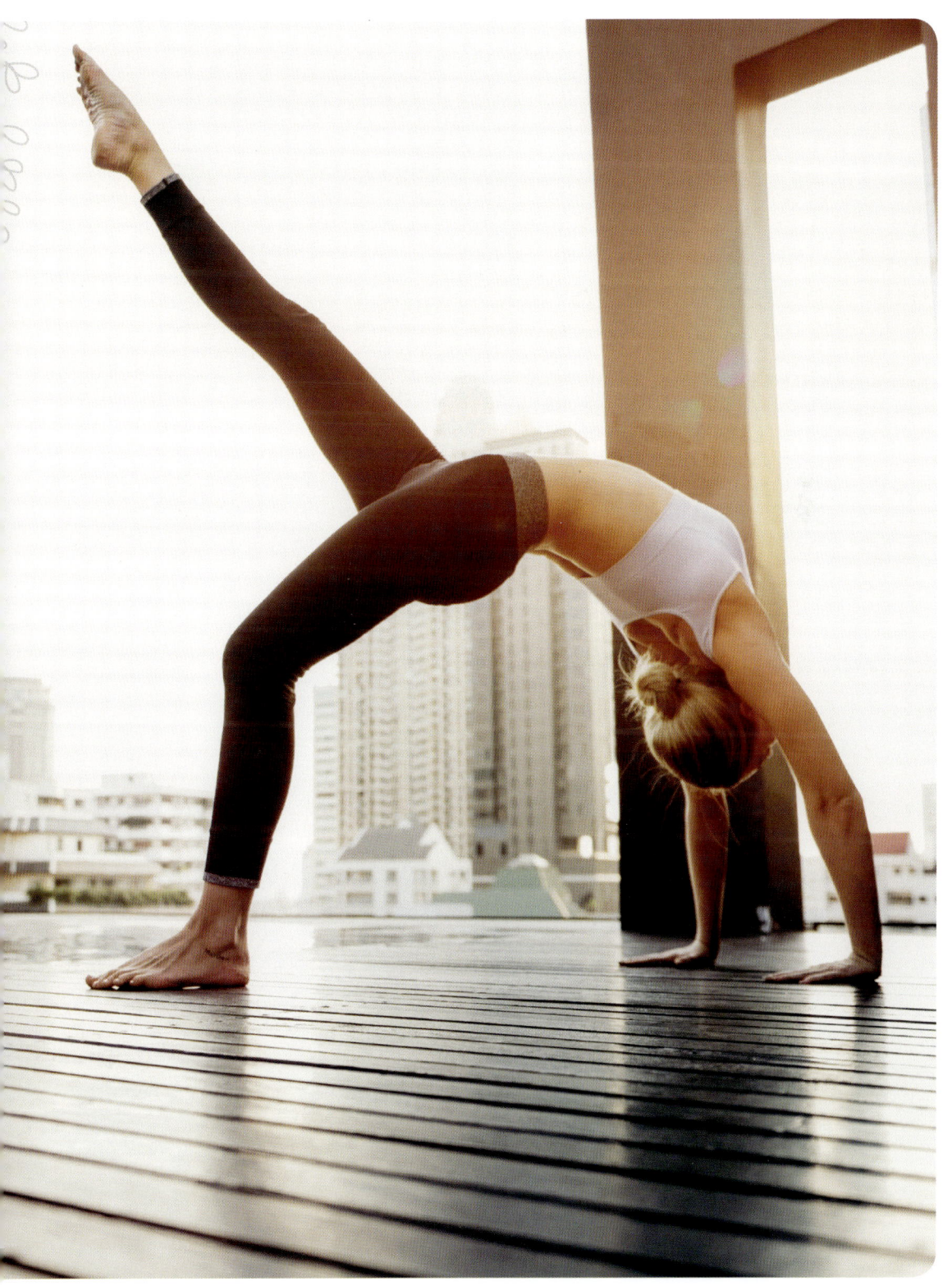

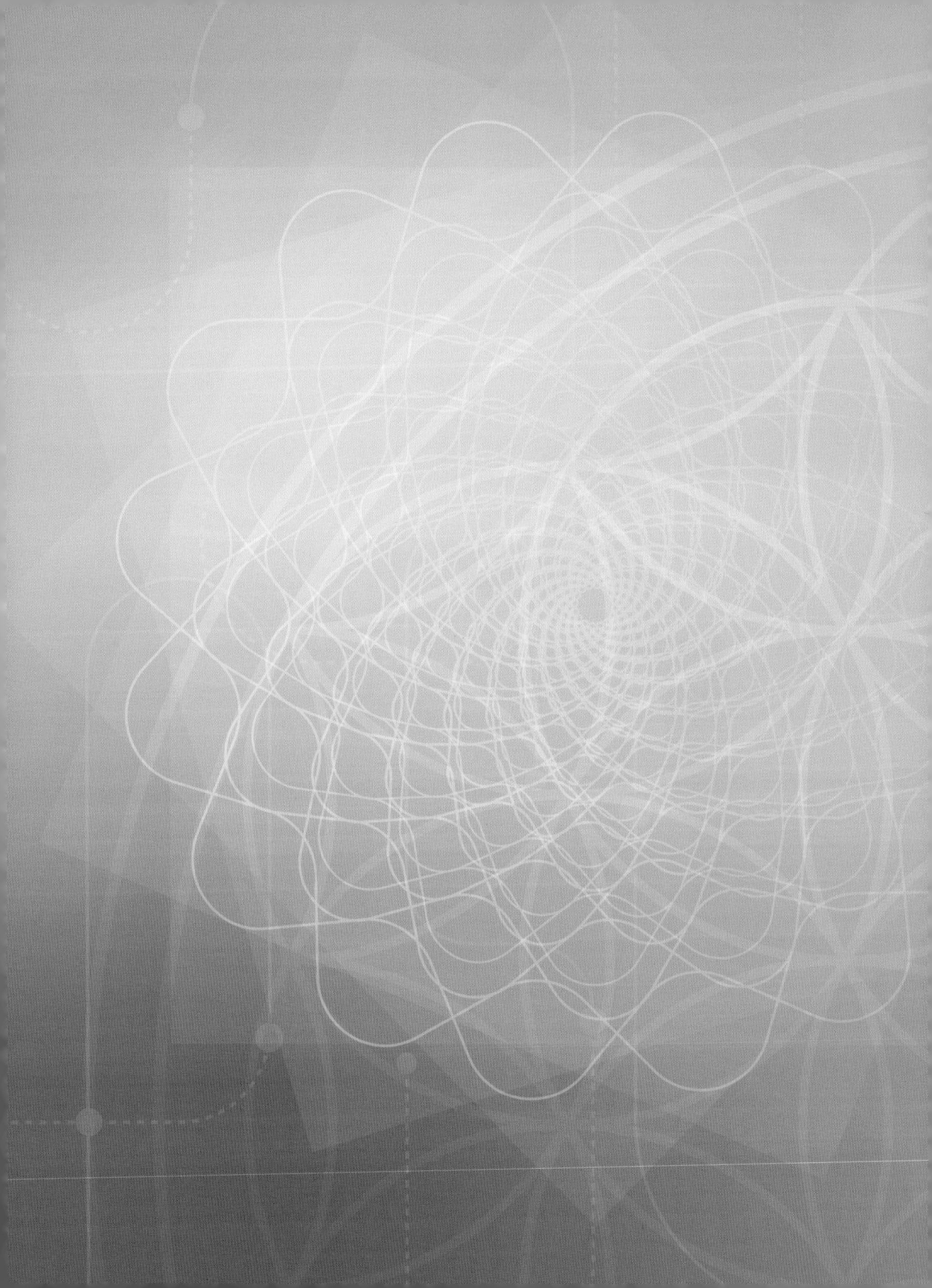

2

THE WEB OF LIGHT

OUR ANCESTORS WERE AWARE OF A WEB OF ENERGY THAT CONNECTS AND INTERPENETRATES ALL THINGS. THE *RIG VEDA*, A SACRED HINDU TEXT, DESCRIBES THE ORIGIN OF THIS ENERGY:

BEFORE THE BEGINNING OF CREATION, NOT EVEN NOTHING EXISTED THEN, NO AIR YET, NOR A HEAVEN. AS THE EXISTENCE OF NOTHING EXPLODED INTO SOMETHING, THE STUFF BETWEEN THE NOTHING WAS BORN.

FIELD OF SACRED ENERGY

Scientists once believed that the space between objects was empty. The German-born physicist Albert Einstein (1879–1955), best known for his two theories of relativity, accepted the idea that the space between objects was empty but had great difficulty in believing it. Unfortunately, the scientific instruments available during Einstein's lifetime weren't powerful enough to measure very subtle energy, so the experiments he carried out to determine whether or not space was empty suggested that it was. This posed two questions, which were difficult to answer. First, if space was indeed empty, what kept the objects contained within it apart? Second, how did light and sound travel, because without energy waves to carry them we would live in a dark and soundless world.

More recently, with the advent of increasingly sophisticated scientific instruments, scientists in the United States have been able to record an extremely subtle energy that permeates all space and interconnects with all objects in the universe. This energy field has been named 'the web of light' and 'the Divine Matrix', and in esoteric circles it's known as the 'ether'. Ether is the accumulation of energies that stores everything that has ever occurred since the birth of the universe. In the physical body, ether is stored in the DNA. This 'cellular' memory contains a record of every experience we've had in our many lifetimes on Earth. These records of our past, present and future are known as the akashic records, from the Sanskrit word *akasa*, meaning 'sky'. All of us have a right to access these but can only do so with the help of our spiritual guides.

According to Gregg Braden in his book *The Divine Matrix*, learning to access this field enables us to create the things that we need in this life and can bring about instantaneous healing. Braden believes that the two most important ingredients for accessing this field are our thoughts and emotions. If we have a physical problem, for example, we have to believe that we're already healed and also feel the joy that healing brings.

The web in action

We can compare this web of light that permeates the universe to a spider's web. When a fly becomes entangled in the spider's web, it sends a vibration along the strands of the web, informing the spider that its dinner has arrived. Similarly, what we think and feel sends along the strands of the web of light vibrational frequencies that can affect people, countries and world situations. Have you ever wondered how sometimes, when the phone rings, you intuitively know who the

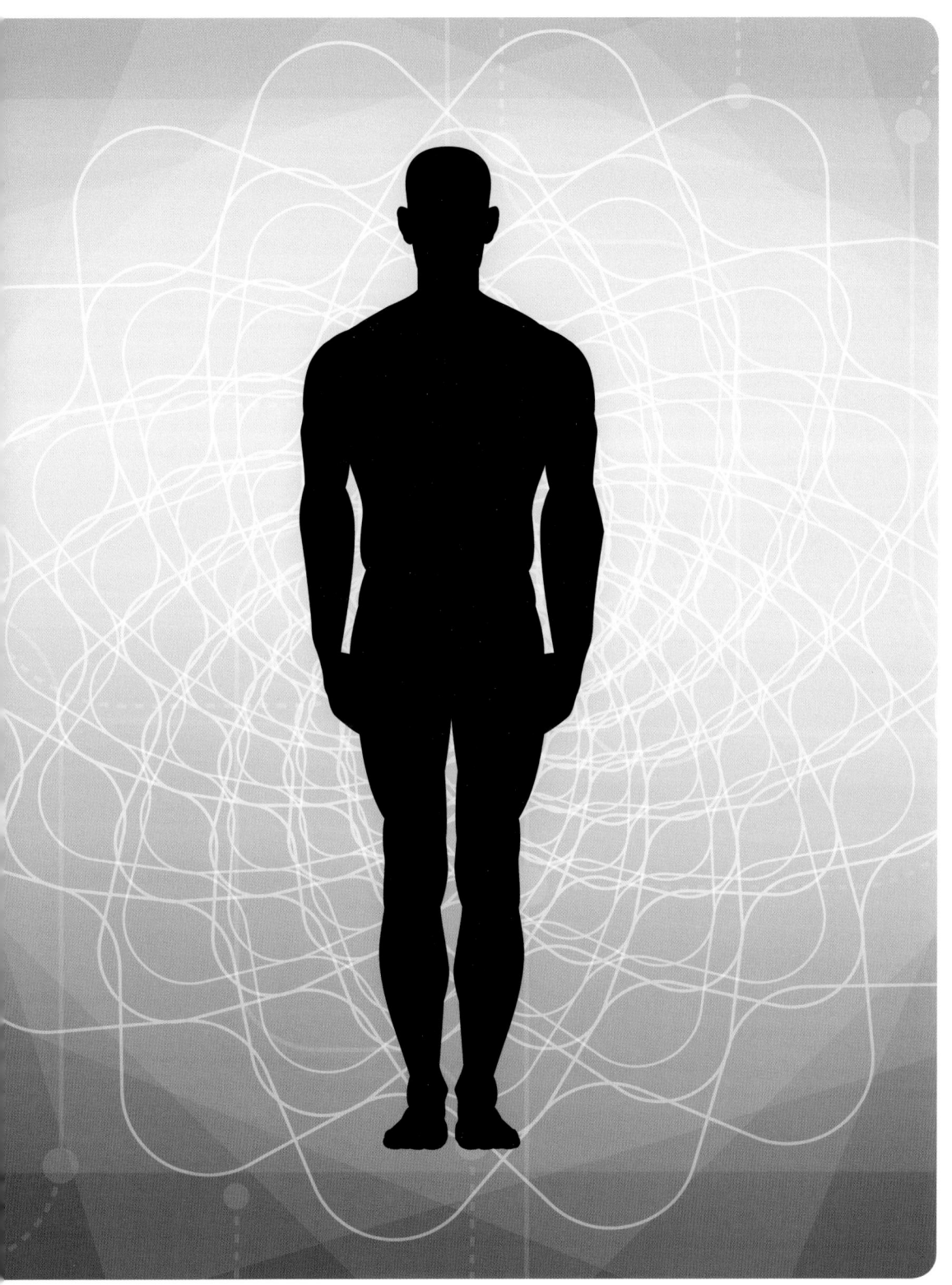

caller is before you answer the call? If we apply the web of light theory here, then we can say that the caller, in thinking about you prior to dialling your number, creates with their thoughts an energy frequency that, as it travels to you along the web, you intuitively pick up. The same theory applies to days of prayer for world peace, where countries that are the subject of prayers may experience reduced levels of violence and crime. This is one of the reasons why yoga puts such great emphasis on the power of positive thinking. As we've already seen in Chapter 1, the first yama is non-violence, and this applies not only to our actions but also to our thoughts.

Yoga students are asked to be aware at various times during the day of what they're thinking. When they become aware of negative thought patterns, they're asked to reverse these to positive ones. They're also reminded that watching violence in the form of films or computer games tends to encourage violence. Perhaps every day we should remind ourselves of that wonderful prayer of St Francis of Assisi:

Lord, make me an instrument of Thy peace:
Where there is hatred, let me sow love;
Where there is injury, pardon;
Where there is doubt, faith;
Where there is despair, hope;
Where there is darkness, light;
Where there is sadness, joy.

O Divine Master, grant that I may not so much seek
To be consoled as to console,
To be understood as to understand,
To be loved, as to love,
For it is in giving that we receive,
It is in pardoning that we are pardoned,
And it is in dying that we are born to eternal life.

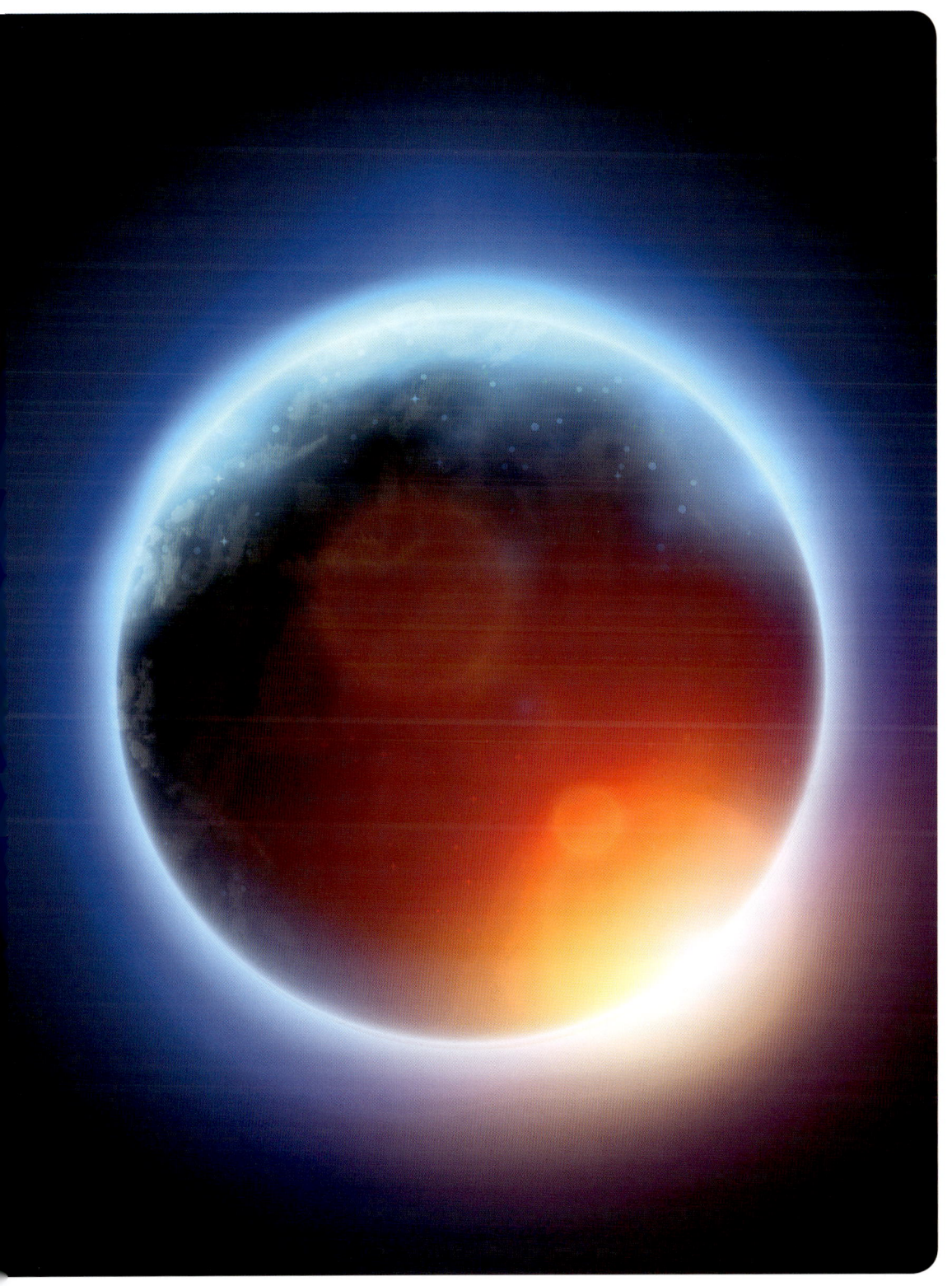

The biologist Bruce Lipton in his book *The Biology of Belief* emphasizes that we're co-creators with the creator and so create our own reality with our thoughts and feelings. Many of the enlightened beings that have walked the Earth knew how to achieve this. For example, devotees of the Indian spiritual master Sai Baba witnessed him materializing objects out of space, and the Christ carried out spontaneous healings. All such masters knew the web of light and how to work with it.

The power of thought

It has long been accepted that our DNA is the fundamental genetic material of all cells, and is present in the nucleus of the cell, where it forms part of the chromosome and acts as the carrier of genetic information. It has therefore also been accepted that if specific diseases are passed on to us through our DNA, the likelihood of us contracting those diseases is great. However, recent research carried out by physicists has shown that our DNA can be switched on and off by our thoughts and emotions.

Until recently, it was also believed that the nucleus was the brain of the cell. But experiments where the nucleus has been removed from the cell have shown that the cell continues to breathe, take in nutrients and excrete waste. The only function that the cell was unable to perform was to divide. Physicists then went on to research which part of the cell was its brain. They discovered that the brain was contained in the shell surrounding each cell, and it was this shell that responded to light, sound and thought. With this new information, surely we should start to watch what we're thinking and to surround ourselves with harmonious rather than discordant sounds. Perhaps we should reflect on these matters and contemplate how we can change the way in which we think and work in order to return to a state of peace, balance and harmony.

The shape of light

In sacred geometry, the solid figure related to the ether, the subtle energy that surrounds all objects, is the dodecahedron. This solid has twelve faces, each of which is a pentagram, one of the most potent sacred symbols. When correctly drawn, the pentagram has four points forming a square and the fifth point in mid-heaven. To some extent, it's the symbol of man, with the two lower points representing the feet, the two middle points the arms and the upper point the head. The pentagram is thought to be the shape in which the universe is contained. Our bodies are also thought to be contained within a pentagram. If this notion is accepted, we could say that, as the web of light surrounds and interpenetrates the universe, so our own bodies are surrounded and penetrated by their own personal web of light. We might then argue that our personal web of light is derived from the nadis, the subtle energy channels through which prana (the life force or vital energy) flows and contained within the etheric layer of the aura (see Chapter 3). In this case, is it feasible that our personal web of light is responsible for the formation of the triangles of light felt and 'seen' while holding certain asanas? I believe that this is so.

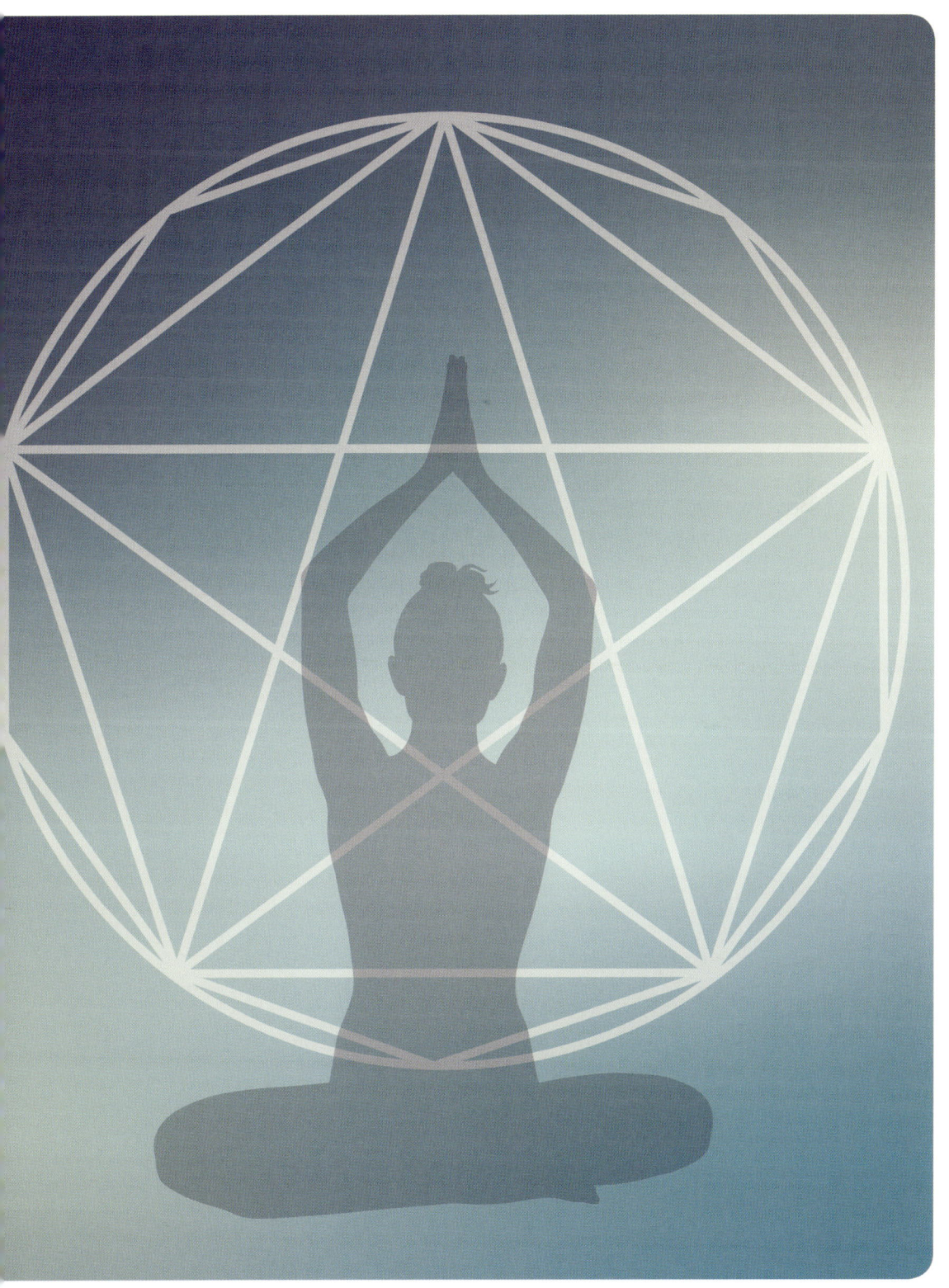

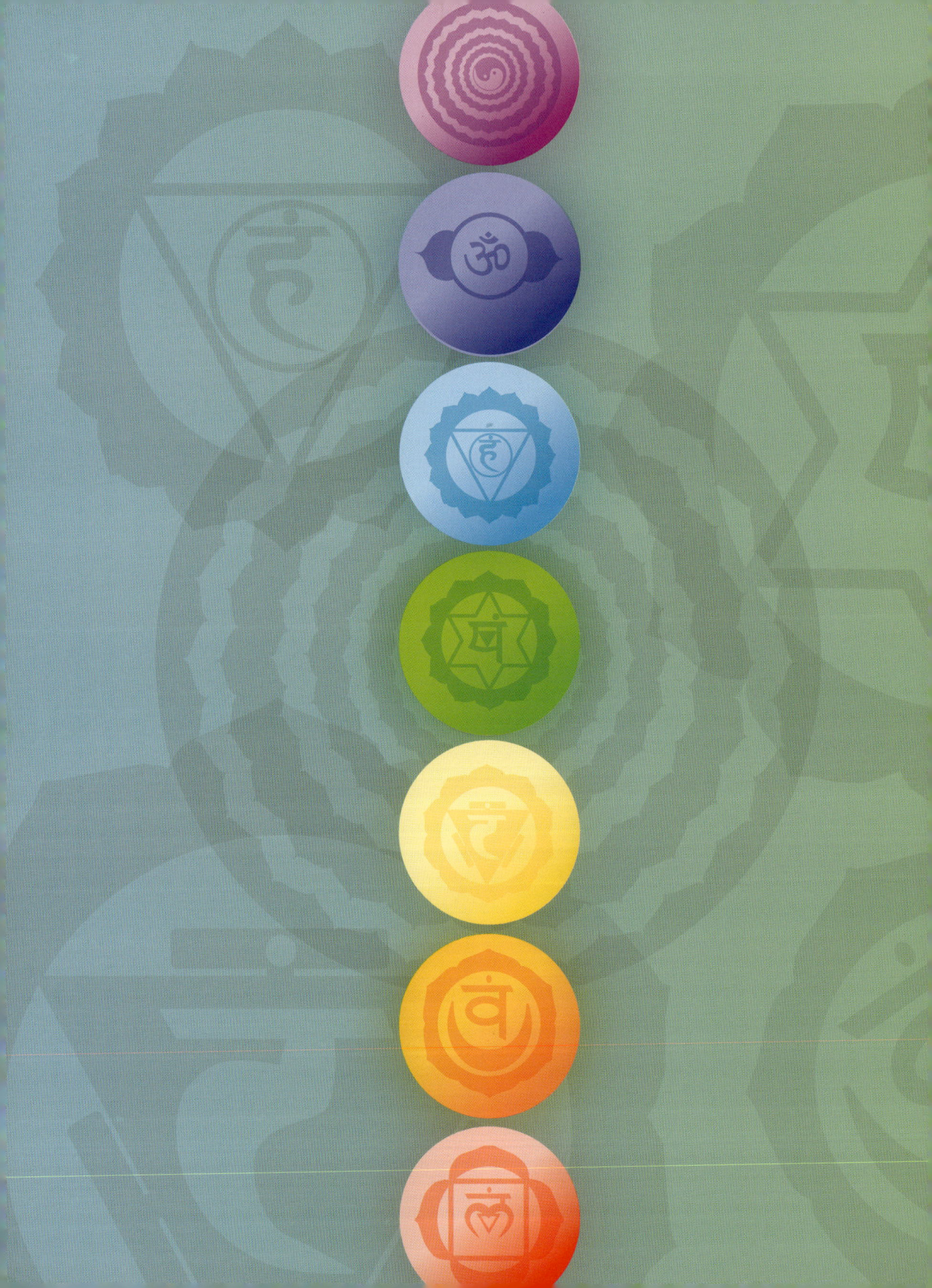

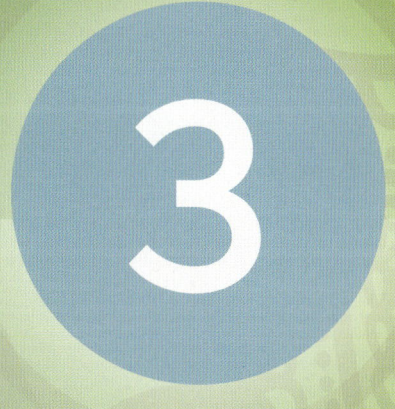

THE CHAKRAS

TO UNDERSTAND AND WORK WITH THE
TRIANGLES OF LIGHT PRESENT IN THE BODY
AND IN THE ELECTROMAGNETIC FIELD THAT
SURROUNDS IT, WE FIRST NEED TO APPRECIATE
THE FUNCTION OF THE AURA AND THE TEN
MAJOR, AND TWENTY-ONE MINOR, CHAKRAS.

INTO THE LIGHT

The chakras are centres of light formed by the intersection of the nadis. A major chakra is formed where twenty-one nadis intersect, a minor chakra where fourteen nadis intersect and an acupuncture point where seven nadis intersect. It's these chakras, or centres of light, that are instrumental in forming the majority of the light triangles.

Seeing triangles

The first step towards generating the triangles is to visualize the triangle while holding the posture. There's a very subtle difference between visualization and imagination. Visualization is actually seeing the triangle with our inner sight. Imagination is simply picturing the triangle of light, although this eventually leads to visualization. With dedicated practice, you'll feel the triangles first as heat, and they'll then appear before your inner sight as brilliant white triangles of light. The creation of these triangles forms part of our soul's evolution, and bringing them into being involves regular practice of breathing exercises, postures and meditation, together with attention to diet.

Preparing the body

When you practise an asana, the longer you're able to maintain the posture the greater its effect in activating the chakra, or chakras, it works with. The body must, however, be correctly positioned, otherwise the posture's effect upon the chakra is minimal. If you're new to yoga, you may find some of the postures difficult. Start with the easy warming-up movements and, with practice and patience, as your body becomes more supple, you'll gradually be able to move further into a posture.

Working with the chakras through asanas helps to clear them of the accumulated debris of many lifetimes – and clearing chakras is essential if we're to return to our true state as beings of light. Each of the major chakras works with one of our hormone-secreting endocrine glands, therefore bringing our hormonal system into balance, which in turn helps to bring our physical body to optimal health.

THE AURA

The electromagnetic field, or aura, that surrounds each human is ovoid in shape – like an egg standing on its narrower end. The largest part of the aura lies around the head and the smallest around the feet. The aura is filled with constantly changing colours, determined by our thoughts, feelings and general health. It's also full of light triangles, which, I believe, form our personal web, the microcosm of the light web that connects all things present in the universe.

THE SEVEN LAYERS OF THE AURA

The aura consists of seven sheaths or layers. Each layer is slightly larger than the previous layer, but they all interpenetrate each other.

The first layer is the most familiar. It's the physical body that we're able to see, touch and experience.

The second layer of the aura, the one nearest the physical body, is known as 'the etheric double' and is the physical body's blueprint. The etheric double is filled with nadis, the fine energy channels through which prana, or life force, flows. Prana originates from the sun, so on a bright sunny day it's in copious supply and can be seen floating in the atmosphere as minute specks of brilliant white light. On a grey, dull day the amount of prana is diminished. At night, prana is almost non-existent, and at this time we utilize our daytime store.

The nadis are closely linked to our nervous system. As we learnt on the previous page, the intersection of seven nadis creates an acupuncture point, the intersection of fourteen creates a minor chakra and the intersection of twenty-one creates a major chakra. Five of the ten major chakras are situated in line with the spine, the sixth is between the eyebrows, the seventh on top of the head, the eighth at the medulla oblongata (roughly the base of the skull), the ninth around 15 cm (6 in) above the head and the tenth about the same distance below the feet.

The base chakra, located at the coccyx, is where two of the three major nadis originate. These nadis are known as the ida and pingala. The ida nadi sits on the left side of the body and is the negative strand. It's associated with the moon, coolness and the right hemisphere of the brain. It also relates to the path of consciousness and psychic unfoldment, and is connected to the parasympathetic nervous system. Pingala

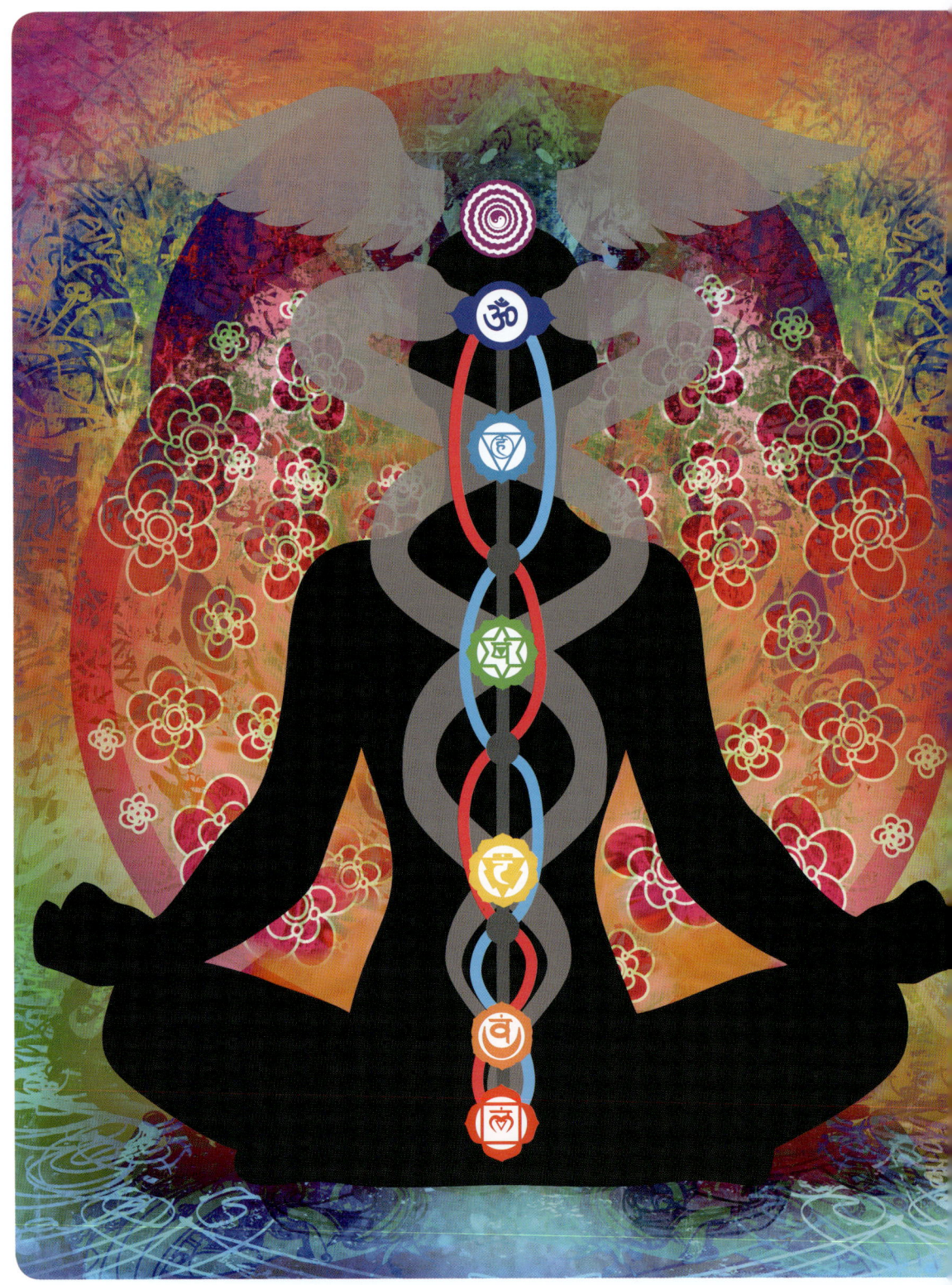

is the positive strand channelling the dynamic energy of prana. It's associated with the right side of the body and with the sun, heat, the left hemisphere of the brain and the sympathetic nervous system. The two nadis entwine around the lower chakras in clockwise and anticlockwise directions, forming figures of eight, until they end at the brow chakra. These nadis are sometimes symbolized as a black and white snake, representing our dual nature. To reach the state of enlightenment, this duality has to be integrated into wholeness – symbolized by the two nadis meeting at the brow chakra.

The third major nadi, the sushumna, is situated inside the spinal column, and extends from the base chakra to the brow chakra, passing through the four major chakras in between. The sushumna houses two additional nadis, vajra and chitrini, which are enclosed within each other to form the tube that carries the 'kundalini' energy. The kundalini is the union of three fires – electric fire, solar fire and fire by friction – chanelled by the ida, pingala and sushumna nadis, respectively.

The third layer of the aura is our astral or emotional body. In a number of people I've worked with, this layer is the one that vibrates to the wrong frequency. The causes are often emotional turmoil and an area of conditioning that the person is afraid to look at and change. Because all the layers of the aura interpenetrate, if any one layer resonates to the wrong frequency, the entire aura will be affected. Consider what happens when you're trying to find the solution to a difficult situation. Thinking hard and long about the problem causes a certain amount of emotional unrest, and if this can't be resolved it's felt as nervous tension in the physical body, which then manifests as a form of digestive disorder. The physical body can be seen as a mirror reflecting what's happening to us at an emotional, mental and spiritual level.

The fourth layer is the mental layer. Every thought is an accumulation of energy, expressed as a shape or form, and these thought forms dwell in this fourth layer. As we think of a person or place, we project thought forms towards them. On a positive level (the only level on which we should be operating), this is how absent healing works. There's a lovely story about this, concerning the Buddha. One day, he was sitting in contemplation, when he became aware of arrows of hate projected towards him. When they neared the Buddha's aura, he turned the arrows into beautiful roses before sending them back to their source – a loving and compassionate response to someone who was actively wishing him harm.

On a less conscious level, like tends to attract like, so if we're positive, we'll attract similar positive thoughts. If our thoughts are negative, we'll attract negativity. This again points to the fact that, at some level, we create our own reality.

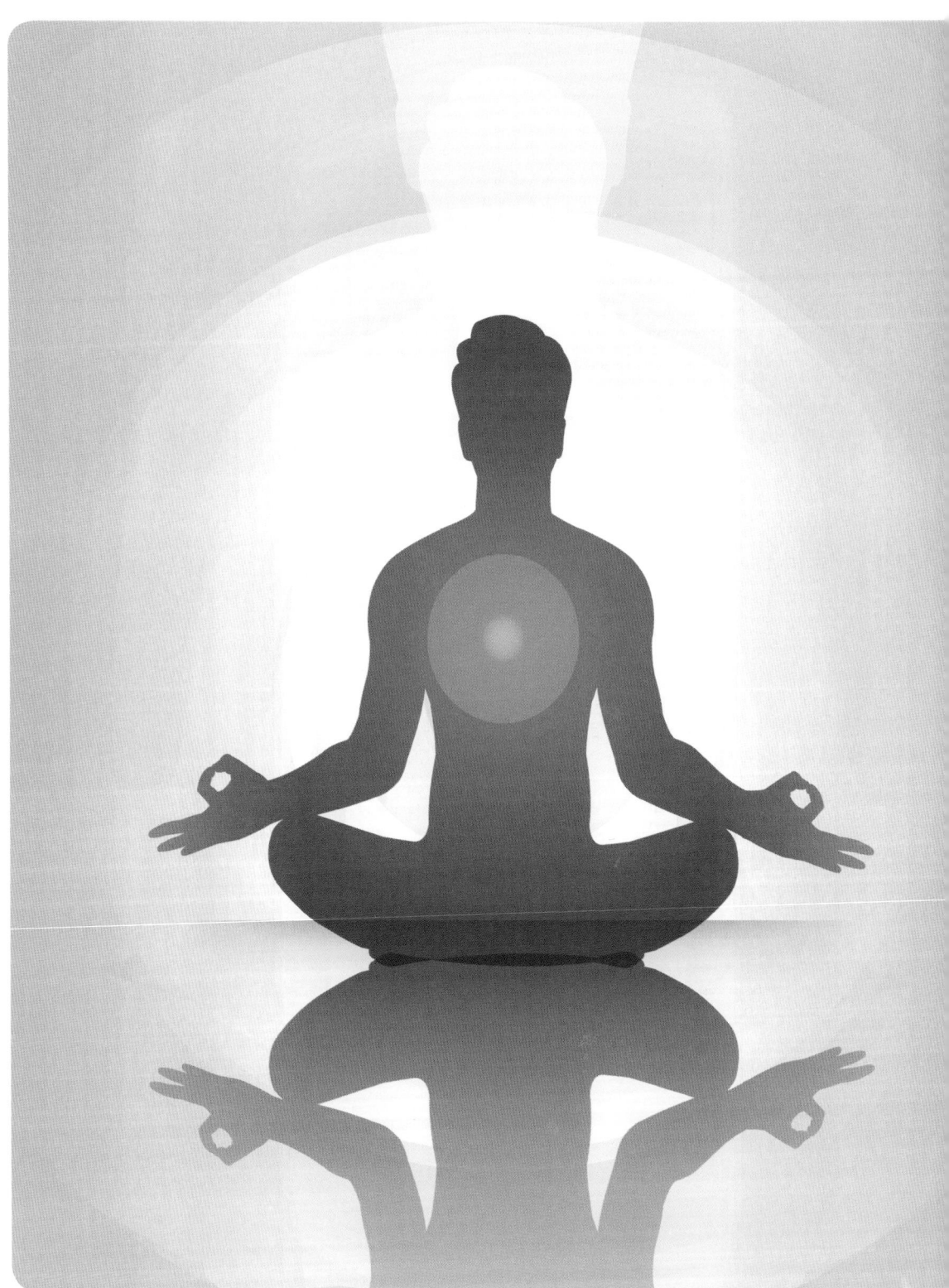

The fifth layer of the aura is the higher mental body. Here lies the source of our intuition. As we evolve through our spiritual practices, we learn to 'hear' and trust our intuition. Working solely with the intellect can lead us into wrong action, but using our intuition, which is, I believe, the voice of our true self, can put us right. Haven't you had times when you've intuitively felt that a course of action, bizarre though it might seem, was right? And following this intuition, haven't you found the course of action to be the correct one, and that subsequent events fell neatly into place? As we evolve spiritually, hearing and obeying our intuition becomes much easier.

The sixth layer of the aura is the causal body, as it houses the cause for our present incarnation. When a soul is ready to incarnate, it chooses the family and country that will provide the conditions needed for its further evolution, and so enable it to pay off some of the karma it has accumulated. Karma is the law of cause and effect. In yoga, it's summarized as 'whatever good you do will be repaid with good, whatever evil, retribution will follow'. The Christ reiterated this when He said: 'As you sow, so shall you reap'. In his book *Conversations with God*, the spiritual teacher Neale Donald Walsh states that whatever situation we find ourselves in, at some level we have created it for ourselves.

The seventh layer – also the largest – is known as 'the bodiless body'. Here the essence of our being resides, our true self, the divine part of us that has neither beginning nor end. It's this part of the self that we aim to discover, and become integrated with, through our yoga practice. This discovery is the final goal of all spiritual paths. In yoga it's called samadhi. When we reach this state, the veil of illusion is dissolved and we radiate the light of our true self.

THE MAJOR CHAKRAS

The eight major chakras (including the alta major chakra, at the base of the skull) associated with and linked to the physical body can be likened to a spiritual ladder (see opposite). Each of these chakras carries a great deal of symbolism, some of which, particularly that relating to the deity residing in them, is thought to have been introduced through Hinduism. While simplified chakra illustrations have been included in this book, the descriptions on the following pages outline the traditional associations symbolized by each chakra and featured on some of the more elaborate depictions. (For further information on this, please see *Chakra Workbook* by Pauline Wills.)

The deities symbolize the qualities needed for the cleansing and revitalizing of their specific chakra. As we evolve spiritually, the chakras are cleansed of old debris and start to expand, bringing balance and healing to the physical body. On this physical level, the chakras are associated with our hormone-producing endocrine system, and if any of them aren't functioning to their full potential, then our hormonal system can be affected. To develop the triangles of light, it's necessary to clear the chakras, as they form the root from which the triangles originate. Chakra clearing often involves considering what changes we need to make in our lives to grow spiritually. This takes courage and can, at times, make us feel insecure as we get rid of old, familiar patterns to allow for the formation of new ones.

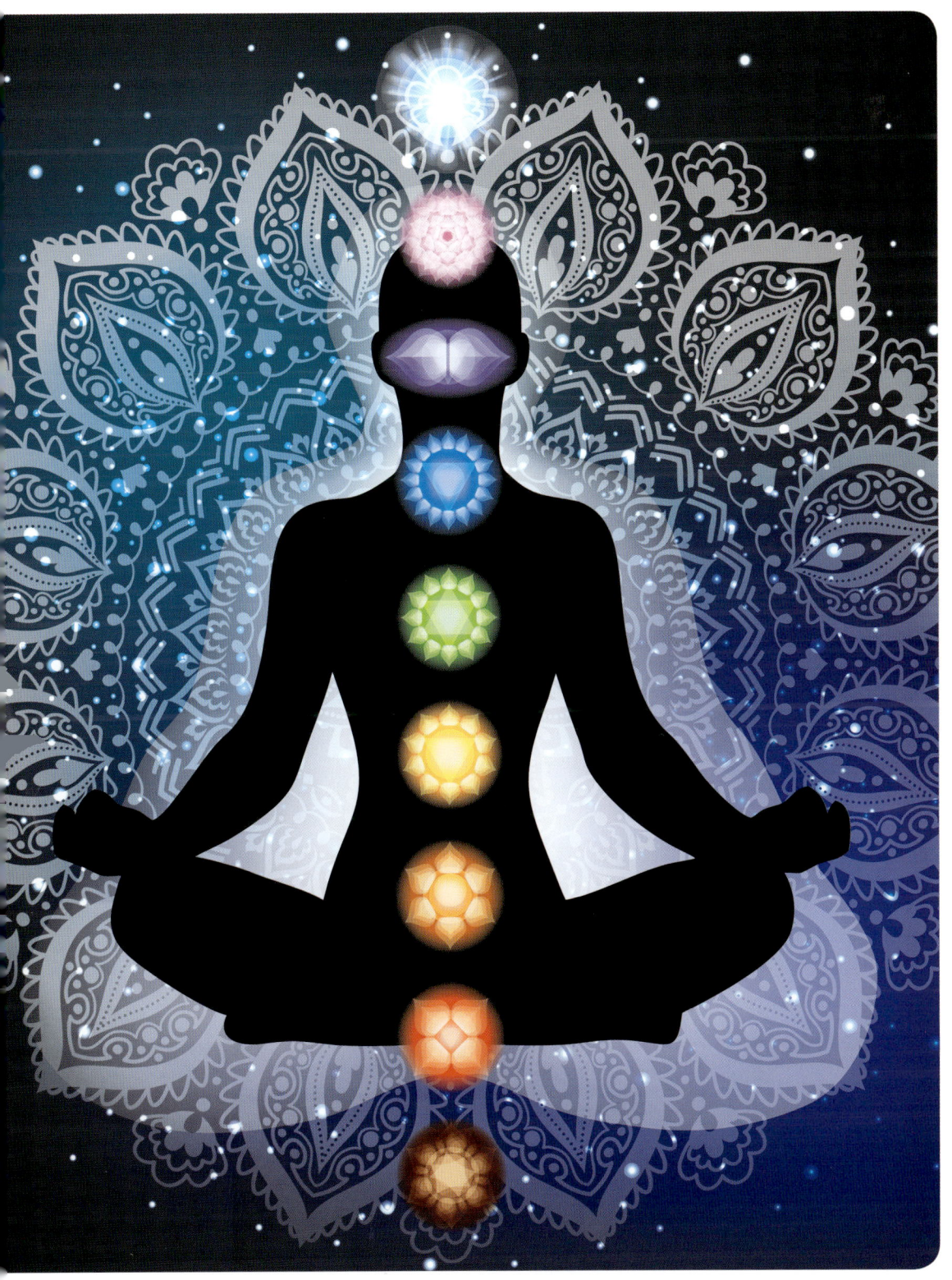

EARTH STAR CHAKRA

Normally depicted as either brown or black, the earth star chakra is about 15–30 cm (6–12 in) below the feet, in line with the spine, and connects with the minor chakra on the sole of each foot. When functioning to its full potential, the earth star chakra allows us to be grounded and centred, and to function effectively on the physical level. It aligns and connects the body to the powerful energies inside the magnetic core of the Earth, helps us to connect with our own energies and those of the Earth and the universe, and is also the grounding point for the rest of our chakra system. It's believed that the earth star chakra holds information on our past lives, the karma we have incurred and the origin of our DNA.

When the earth star chakra is open, we're able to stay fully grounded. It allows those who work as a channel for healing to release any negativity they may have absorbed from their clients. When this chakra is balanced, we feel connected to our inner powers. When it's unbalanced, we could suffer eating disorders, experience problems with feet, legs and hips, and have a poor circulatory system.

BASE CHAKRA

The Sanskrit name for the base chakra is muladhara – *mula* meaning 'root' and *dhara* meaning 'base' or 'support'. The chakra is found at the end of the coccyx, and is depicted as a circle with four outer red petals. A yellow square, often surrounded by eight shining spears, is inside the circle. The yellow square represents the earth element and, like the Earth, is a solid foundation for an aspirant starting their spiritual journey. The spears signify the eight points of the compass, the eight steps of yoga laid down by the sage Patanjali, and the many paths that can be taken towards the state of enlightenment. The mantra or sound associated with this chakra is 'lam'. The associated deities are Indra, Brahman and Dakini, and the symbolic animal is the elephant Airavata. He's shown with seven trunks, representing the seven spectral colours and the seven major planets, and he wears a collar symbolizing our attachment to the Earth and to materialism. The elephant is a slow and heavy animal, attributes that portray some of the qualities of this chakra. Within the triangle that sits within the square lies a phallus, or lingam, around which is coiled the kundalini or serpent power. Above the phallus sits a crescent moon, representing the divine source of all creation.

The base chakra is the seat of one of the physical body's most powerful energies – the kundalini. At a certain stage in an aspirant's spiritual development, this great force rapidly rises through the sashumna nadi, piercing and opening all the major chakras and bringing about a state of enlightenment. Raising this energy prematurely can be extremely dangerous and is not something to experiment with.

Closely connected to our physical body, the base chakra is our centre of survival, giving us the instinct to provide warmth, nourishment and shelter for the body to keep it healthy and strong. It's also our earth-linked chakra, keeping us grounded. Working with the base chakra helps us to realize that we create our own reality, and that if we visualize the things we need for our health and survival, they'll be provided; but with this realization must also come trust and a positive attitude to life.

When the muladhara chakra is balanced, it centres and grounds the physical body, provides it with vitality and makes a person sexually affectionate. Lack of energy here can create depression and a lack of aims in life. An overabundance of the base energy can make a person domineering, aggressive and egoistic. The endocrine glands associated with this chakra are the testes. Some of the physical symptoms that could manifest when the base chakra isn't functioning to its full potential are haemorrhoids, testicular disorders, spinal and leg problems and inhibited rejuvenation of blood cells.

SACRAL CHAKRA

The Sanskrit name for this chakra is svadisthana, meaning 'your abode'. It's situated just below the navel and is shown as a circle with six outer orange petals. Inside the circle is a crescent moon symbolic of female receptivity and the water element. Lying inside the crescent moon is a makara, a legendary animal similar to an alligator and bearing characteristics of a fish, a crocodile and an elephant. The symbolic deities are Varuna, associated with the water element, Vishnu and the goddess Rakini. The mantra to which this chakra resonates is 'vam'.

Water is said to be the liquid counterpart of light and is related to the feminine principle. The element has the power to dissolve, abolish, purify and regenerate, is associated with our emotions and affects the flow of fluids in our physical body. Water flows freely when uninhibited, and one of the challenges of this centre is to see whether we're allowing ourselves to flow freely with the energies of life, or holding on to old emotional patterns that prevent our spiritual evolution. Many men have been conditioned into believing that it's not manly to cry, but holding on to such emotions builds a mighty dam that will eventually break and manifest as a physical ailment.

The sacral chakra is the body's source of vitality and centre of survival through procreation. It therefore influences our sexual feelings and governs our love–hate relationships. The emotions relating to the undermining of women are stored in this centre. Remember that feminine and masculine energies are complementary, and if they're balanced (each accepting the other as divine) they create wholeness. To be whole, we must each learn to integrate our innate feminine and masculine aspects as we grow through our spiritual practices. For the sacral chakra to function fully, we have to come to terms with any negativity surrounding these issues.

At a physical level, this chakra governs the female reproductive organs, the breasts, the skin and the kidneys. Its associated endocrine glands are the adrenals.

When the sacral chakra is cleared, our intuitive powers are opened and our sensitivity heightened; our sexuality is balanced and we become friendly and optimistic. If the chakra becomes deficient in energy, we can become resentful, distrustful, oversensitive, shy and fearful. An overcharged sacral chakra can make us aggressive, manipulative, obsessed with sex and emotionally explosive.

Some of the physical symptoms that can present if this chakra isn't functioning fully relate to the reproductive organs, intestines, bladder, kidneys, circulation and central nervous system. You might also suffer from migraines, irritability and low energy.

SOLAR PLEXUS CHAKRA

Manipura, meaning 'the jewel in the navel', is the Sanskrit name given to the solar plexus chakra. It's situated just above the navel and is shown as a circle with ten yellow outer petals. The chakra is associated with the sun and the fire element, symbolized within the circle by a red downward-pointing triangle bearing the mark of the swastika on each of its three sides. The swastika is an ancient and complex symbol, and in this chakra it represents the fire god Agni and fire's association with life and movement. The deities present are Rudra, Lakini and Vahini. The animal depicted is the ram, connected to the sacred fire of Agni, and the sound is 'ram'.

All nadis are said to originate from the navel, making manipura a centre of power, and also a centre of vitality in the psychic and physical bodies. This is where prana (the upward-flowing vitality) and apana (the downward-flowing vitality) meet, generating the heat necessary to support life. When the two energies unite, the centre wakes – but this can't happen until the traits of the two lower chakras are worked through.

Manipura is linked with the emotional and astral body, and it's where we experience fear, worry and anxiety. It's also the area where we pick up the emotions of others and from which people whose own energies are depleted can withdraw their energy, either consciously or unconsciously. It's important, therefore, for sensitives, psychics and healers to protect this centre.

For manipura to open, allowing us to rise to the heart chakra, we need to work at eradicating all negativity from our life. This is sometimes referred to as walking through the fire of purification. Fear is the most negative of the emotions, because it encases us in a dark grey mist that's hard to penetrate. Some of the challenges we meet as we pursue our chosen path are given to enable us to overcome our fears.

In the physical body, manipura influences our digestive organs, liver, gall bladder, duodenum and pancreas. The associated endocrine glands are the islets of Langerhans, which form part of the pancreas. Some of the physical symptoms that can arise from an imbalance in this chakra are low vitality, liver problems, hypoglycaemia, diabetes, stomach and digestive problems, and muscular and nervous tension.

When the energy of manipura is balanced, we're cheerful, outgoing, spontaneous, relaxed and uninhibited, and respect ourselves and others. We also enjoy good food and physical activity, and show emotional warmth. Excessive energy here can turn us into workaholics and perfectionists, or make us judgemental and resentful of authority. If depleted in this energy, we might suffer from depression, insecurity and fear.

HEART CHAKRA

The Sanskrit name given to this chakra is anahata, which means 'the unstruck' or 'unbeaten sound'. Striking objects together, which sets up vibrations or waves, produces all sound in the universe. The primordial sound, which comes from beyond this universe, is the source of all sound and is known as the anahata sound.

Anahata chakra is situated near the fifth thoracic vertebra and is depicted as a circle with twelve outer green petals. Inside the circle is a smoky blue hexagram made from upward-pointing and downward-pointing triangles. The upward-pointing triangle is red and represents solar energy, fire and masculine energy; it stands for humankind's higher nature, and thus links to our spiritual energies. The downward-pointing triangle is white and is associated with the moon, water, feminine energy, earth energies and the lower nature of mankind. These two triangles are formed in light, through and around the physical body, and their interlacing characterizes the union of opposites: 'as above, so below'.

The heart chakra is our point of balance and lies central to the three upper and three lower chakras. If we were to draw a horizontal line through these six chakras, and then separate the three upper and three lower with a horizontal line, it would create a cross, symbolizing all aspects of the self. Anahata is the cross's centre, where our spiritual and earth energies meet, and is connected to the duality of our nature and to wholeness. Any path we care to journey along challenges us to look at and accept our dual nature, so that we might balance and then transcend this duality to achieve wholeness. This involves, for example, accepting our male and female aspects, our good and bad sides, our intellect and creativity. We must experience opposites in order to understand and appreciate them. If we never experienced the bad, we wouldn't appreciate the good; if we were never ill, we wouldn't appreciate feeling well. Life is based on experience, and our ultimate challenge is to integrate all our life experiences into a state of wholeness or oneness with the supreme intelligence behind creation.

The deities present in the heart chakra are: Vayu – god of the air element and master of the chakra's mantra 'yam'; Ishu – another form of Shiva, the Lord of the Dance, and overlord to the three lower chakras; and the goddess Kakini. The animal depicted is the antelope. Anahata chakra is also linked to the air element and the sense of touch.

This is the centre where we experience love in all its many aspects, and it's here that we connect with those we love. The ultimate expression of love is an unconditional love, which doesn't judge, or demand expectations from, the people with whom we come into contact. However, to love others unconditionally we first have to love all aspects of ourselves. Many of us are conditioned into thinking that loving ourselves is selfish, which is far from the truth. To love our physical body is to respect the vehicle in which our true self dwells. In doing this, we try to keep our body in optimum health by being aware of the kind of food we eat and our general lifestyle. In loving our thoughts and feelings, we're able to detect any changes that aren't conducive to our well-being.

Anahata chakra influences the heart and lungs, the immune and circulatory systems and the lymph glands. The endocrine gland with which it's associated is the thymus. Anahata is linked to our mental body, which gives it its polarity of thought coming in and thought going out. When we transcend this polarity, we transcend the mind to connect with divine love.

When the heart chakra's energies are balanced, we feel compassionate, have a desire to nurture others and are able to practise unconditional love. A well-balanced anahata makes a person friendly, outgoing and in touch with their own feelings. A lack of energy here can create paranoia, indecisiveness, a fear of rejection and of being hurt, and a need for constant reassurance. In excess, this energy can create depression, and make a person moody, demanding, over-critical, possessive and adept at conditional love.

A malfunctioning heart chakra can be responsible for breathing and lung problems, asthma, high blood pressure and heart disease.

THROAT CHAKRA

The Sanskrit name for the throat chakra is visshudha, meaning 'to purify'. The chakra is located at the first cervical vertebra and is symbolized as a circle with sixteen outer blue petals. Inside the circle is a downward-pointing triangle with a white circle at its centre. This circle represents the full moon and symbolizes psychic power.

The throat chakra is associated with the element ether, or akasha, and the sense of hearing. The deities present are Sadasiva, Shakini and Ambara, and the mantra is 'ham'. The animal is the elephant, but at this chakra he no longer wears a collar, showing at this stage of our journey we've been liberated from our bondage to materialism.

In this chakra – our door or bridge to higher levels of consciousness – the four lower elements are refined to their purest essence before being dissolved into the ether. The earth element at the base chakra is dissolved into the water element at the sacral chakra, leaving its essence as the sense of smell. At the solar plexus chakra, the water element is then transformed by the fire element into vapour, and its essence becomes taste. When the fire element enters the heart chakra, it gives movement to the air, and its essence becomes touch. Then when the air unites with the ether at the throat centre, it becomes pure sound.

Sound is sacred in Eastern mysticism, and the throat chakra is linked with sound through music and the spoken word. Every word we utter creates a vibration in the surrounding ether, which, depending on the intent behind each utterance, can be harmful or beneficial. It's also said that the whole of creation was brought into being by sound. The primordial sound, inaudible to the physical ear and conceived to be the origin of all matter and energy in the universe, is 'aum', the mantra belonging to the brow chakra. Because a human being is a microcosm of the macrocosm, every cell that institutes the physical body is also sounding a note. If we're sick, we go out of tune, and in nada yoga (the yoga of sound) mantras are used to bring the body back to a state of wholeness. As we progress along our spiritual path and learn to quieten the constant chatter of the mind, we're able to 'tune in' and hear with our inner ear the harmonies that are created throughout our being.

At a physical level, vishuddha governs our throat, shoulders, the parathyroids and thyroid gland. It's linked with the digestive tract through the oesophagus, with the genital organs through the hormones secreted by the thyroid gland, and with the lungs and bronchial tubes.

When this chakra is balanced, we become centred, contented and a good speaker. We can be musically or artistically inspired and have a leaning towards meditation. If vishuddha is deficient in energy, we can become timid, inconsistent, unreliable, devious, manipulative and afraid of sex. If it's overstimulated, we can become arrogant, self-righteous, dogmatic and an excessive talker.

Some of the physical ills that may arise if this centre isn't functioning to its full potential are digestive and weight problems, thyroid problems, throat infections, headaches and exhaustion.

When the throat chakra is awakened, divine nectar (the mystical elixir of immortality) is tasted. This nectar is a sweet secretion produced by the lalana gland, located near the back of the throat. The gland is stimulated by higher yogic practices and its nectar is reputed to sustain a yogi for any length of time without food or water.

BROW CHAKRA

Ajna, meaning 'to command', is the Sanskrit name for the brow chakra. This centre, located on the forehead, midway between the eyebrows, is sometimes known as the third eye, and it's where we receive information from our higher self via our intuition.

The brow chakra is composed of ninety-six petals but is depicted as a circle with two outer petals of indigo. These petals connect with the right and left lobes of the pituitary gland and represent the combination of our existence's two polarities. They're likewise linked to the right and left hemispheres of the brain. The right hemisphere is the seat of insight, connected with psychic power; the left hemisphere is the seat of intelligence, giving us an overview of the world. At this centre, the three main nadis (ida, pingala and sushumna) unite before ascending to the crown chakra.

At the centre of the chakra is an inverted triangle representing the fundamental triune nature of the Supreme Reality. This trinity encompasses reality, consciousness and joy. Inside the triangle is the mantra 'aum' – the principal Hindu mantra – composed of the three sounds of A (the sound of creation), U (the sound of preservation) and M (the sound of dissolution). Thus, the supreme god Brahma itself is the essence of this all-encompassing mantra, the universal sound. 'Aum' is the sound that's understood to be heard in the most profound silence. It's likened to a flame in its pure radiance – a flame that expands into the white light of consciousness. It's believed that, in the higher states of meditation, this sound can be heard with our inner hearing as it vibrates through the physical body. The deities present in the brow chakra are the goddess Hakini and Shiva in the form of Itara.

The ajna chakra is also known as 'the door' – the door we must go through to make contact with the white light of consciousness. In the Christian scriptures, the Christ said: 'Knock and the door will be opened to you'. We knock at the door of the brow chakra by raising our eyes to the chakra in meditation; and when we're ready and the door opens we experience a deep indigo oval shape with a six-pointed star at its centre, the indigo oval surrounded by golden light. When this centre is functioning to its full potential, our duality is integrated into wholeness and the centre's energy is raised to the crown chakra and to God Consciousness.

On a physical level, the brow chakra is connected to the nervous system, nose, eyes, ears and brain. The associated endocrine gland is the pituitary. When the chakra is functioning to its full potential, we have no fear of death, realizing that death is our passage into the spiritual world. We're not preoccupied with fame or fortune or material possessions. The veil of illusion is pierced and we recognize ourselves as spiritual beings, a tiny part of the whole creation. The gifts of telepathy and astral travel open and we're able to access our past lives. When we open these gifts, it's important not to become attached to them. As my own teacher used to say, there's something far greater beyond them.

If anja is deficient in energy it can make us afraid of success, undisciplined, non-assertive and unable to distinguish between the ego self and the true self. If there's excess energy, it can make us religiously dogmatic, proud, manipulative and obsessed by ego.

Some of the physical symptoms that can arise when this chakra isn't functioning to its full potential are hormonal imbalances, migraines, headaches, catarrh, sinus problems, eye problems and sleeplessness.

CROWN CHAKRA

The Sanskrit name given to the crown chakra is sahasrara, meaning 'a thousandfold'. This chakra, situated at the crown of the head, is regarded as the centre of infinity. Its symbolism is complex and has received many interpretations, all of which point to the attainment of self-realization through our devotion to work and study. These interpretations describe the integrated state of our dual nature and the altered state of consciousness brought about by raising the latent power in the base chakra. Here again I must stress the importance of working slowly with yourself. If this latent energy is raised prematurely, before you're completely ready, you could suffer both physical and psychological damage. The yogi Gopi Krishna, the author of a number of books on yoga, was a great authority on this process. He inadvertently raised the kundalini energy and as a result endured great pain for many years. You should therefore seek the guidance of a teacher who has gained the wisdom to work with this latent energy and to know when you're ready to work with it. I believe that, if we practise our yoga with the right intention and are finally ready to undertake the raising of this powerful energy, the master will appear to guide us on the final stage of our journey.

This, the seventh, chakra is depicted as a thousand-petalled white or pale violet lotus that has its head turned downwards. The petals are arranged in twenty rows, each row of fifty petals containing the fifty letters of the Sanskrit alphabet, written in white. Inside the petals are the circle, the mandala for the full moon and the mandala for the sun. These two mandalas signify the union of our dual nature to wholeness.

The complex symbolism of sahasrara isn't easily understood until we've experienced the void that we have to pass through to unite with our true self. Mystics and seers of all religions who have experienced transcendent states of consciousness have found the experience difficult to describe in comprehensible terms. Often they've resorted to using parables and imagery in their efforts to explain the unexplainable. Imagine how difficult it would be for you to explain, for example, the taste of an orange to someone who has never eaten one. When we reach the state of transcendence, we're free from the wheel of life – the wheel of rebirth – because we've remembered who we truly are, and to be reborn would, therefore, serve no purpose. Those who are filled with an insatiable desire to access higher planes of consciousness will achieve their desire only through intense meditation and self-discipline.

When the crown chakra starts to fully open, we become drawn to mystical teachings. Spirituality is defined through unique individual experience, an inner knowing rather than external dogma. At this stage in our development we may start to see auras, to experience a sense of joyful awe and wonder at the beauty and vastness of creation and to gain an inner understanding of universal truths. When fully opened, this chakra unites with the brow chakra to form the halo depicted around the head of saints and other enlightened beings.

When the crown chakra is blocked, creativity is blocked and we've no sense of our spirituality. We could veer towards extreme materialism and have little interest in anything other than the mundane. We might become involved in fundamentalist religion or ideology.

The physical symptoms that can arise from this chakra include brain disease, migraines and endocrine system disorders. Psychological problems can also arise.

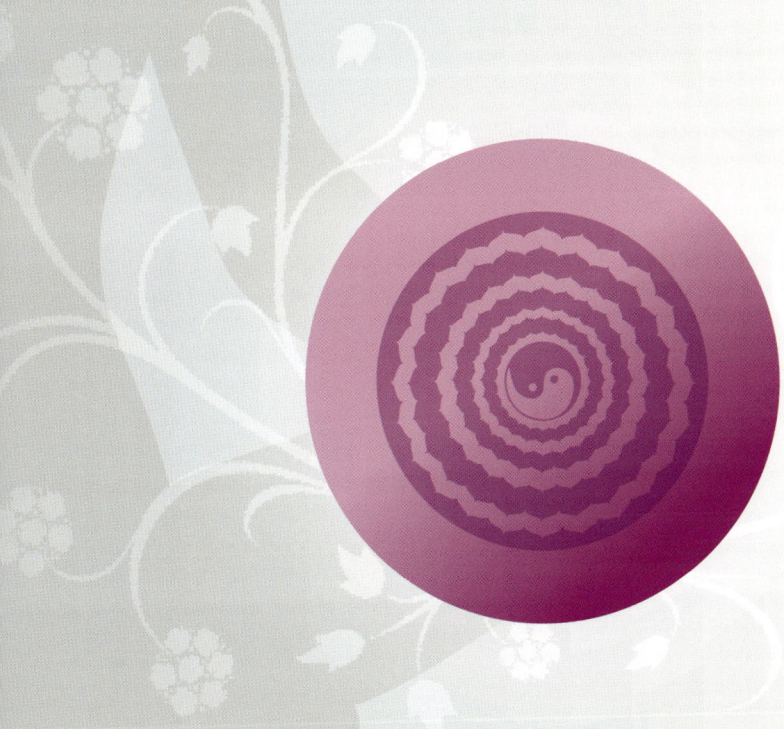

ALTA MAJOR CHAKRA

The alta major chakra is situated at the medulla oblongata, roughly at the base of the skull. It radiates to the colour white but is frequently depicted as magenta. It's connected to the carotid glands, which are small reddish-brown glands on either side of the neck, where the carotid artery divides. Their main function is to ensure an adequate supply of oxygen to the physical body's tissues. Oxygen levels are maintained by a reflex, operating between the carotid gland and the respiratory centre of the brain.

Spiritually, the alta major has a close connection with the brow chakra and the eyes. When we're able to unite these two chakras, they create, together with the physical eyes, a triangle of light that then shines through our eyes – the mirror of the soul.

This chakra is known as 'the mouth of God', because it's where the life force (the breath of God) enters and sustains the physical body. The life force entering the alta major is what sustains mystics who have lived for many years without food or water.

The centre plays an important role in the formation of many of the light triangles present in humans.

SOUL STAR CHAKRA

White in colour, the soul star chakra is located in the aura, approximately 15 cm (6 in) above the crown chakra. Some believe this chakra to be the seat of the soul because it's able to connect our own soul to enlightenment by transferring light to it. The soul star chakra also enhances our relationship with the universe.

Once the chakra is awakened, our soul transcends from our ego self to an enlightened, spiritual, joyful state. The soul star has the very important role of collecting and then transferring cosmic energy to the seven lower chakras, to energize and clear those chakras in readiness for them to fully open. I also feel that the soul star chakra acts as a transformer of energy, transforming the powerful, spiritual light to a frequency that can be tolerated by the physical body, which varies with each individual and is dependent on a person's spiritual awareness. The greater our spiritual awareness, the greater our understanding of the sacred web of light and the triangles that are formed with our own web of light.

If this chakra is unbalanced, symptoms such as headaches, confusion, depression and mental fatigue can appear. When the soul star is balanced, you feel connected to your higher self, contented and ready to see and realize all aspects of life.

MINOR CHAKRAS

Also present in the aura are twenty-one minor chakras, which have a part to play in the formation of some of the light triangles. These minor chakras are connected to various organs throughout the physical body and emit a subtler shade of the colour radiated by the major chakra located nearest to them. The following table shows where these chakras are situated and their associated colour.

Position of minor chakras	Associated colour
One behind each eye	shade of indigo
One at the base of each ear	shade of indigo
One midway along each clavicle	shade of blue
One in the palm of each hand	shade of blue
One near the thymus gland	turquoise
One connected with the nipple of each breast	shade of green
One connected to the liver	shade of yellow
One connected to the stomach	shade of yellow
One connected with the gonads (female ovaries) (male testes)	shade of orange
One behind each knee	shade of red
One on the sole of each foot	shade of red
Two connected with the spleen	shade of orange

The formation of the light triangles depends on these chakras, together with the major chakras. Working to become sensitive to these energy wheels is extremely important.

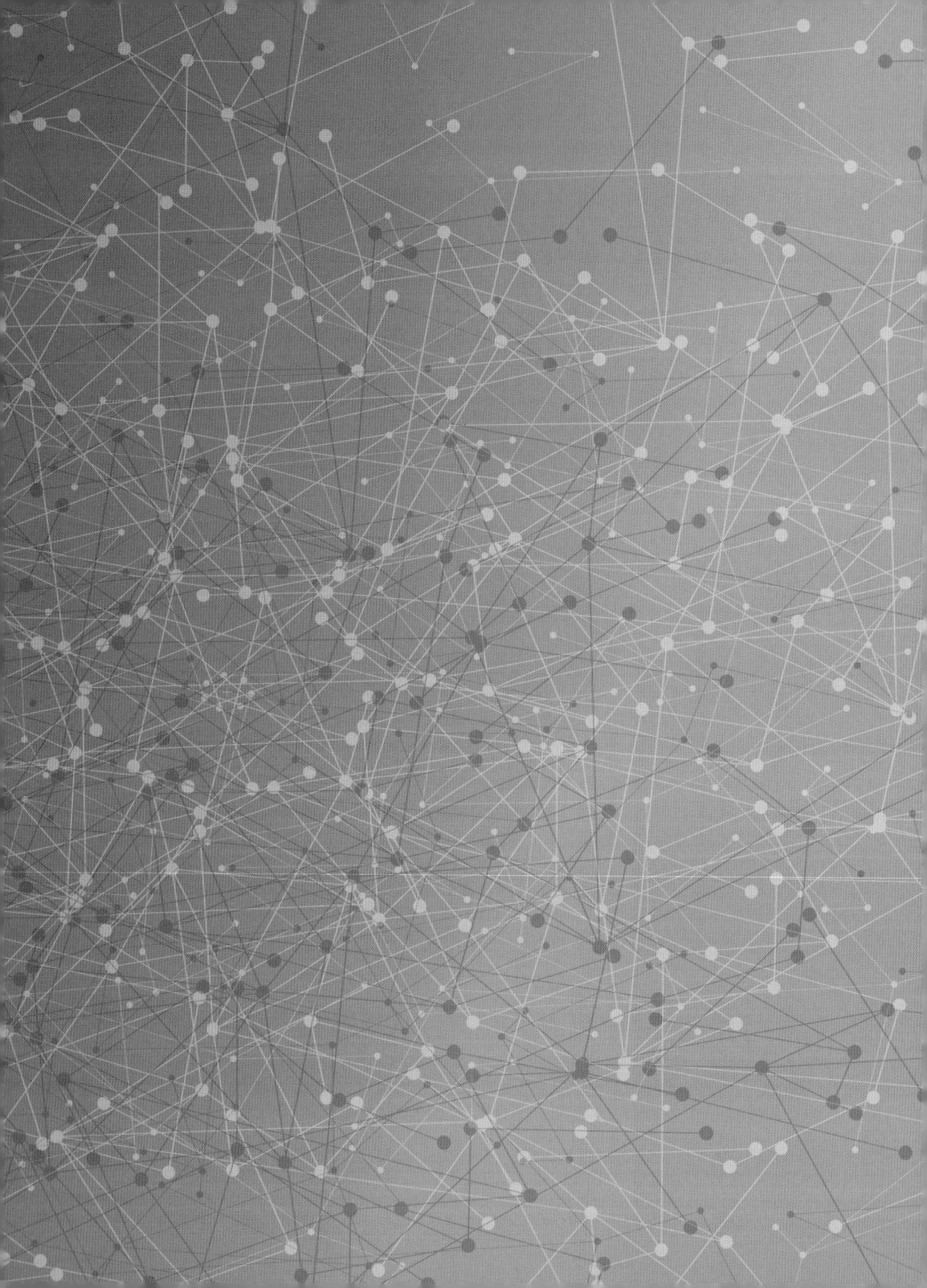

4

PRANAYAMA

PRANA IS THE VITAL FORCE THAT PERVADES THE WHOLE COSMOS. THOUGH CLOSELY RELATED TO THE AIR WE BREATHE, PRANA IS A MORE SUBTLE ENERGY – THE ENERGY ESSENCE WITHIN EVERYTHING IN THE UNIVERSE. PRANAYAMA IS A SERIES OF BREATHING TECHNIQUES THAT STIMULATE AND INCREASE PRANA, AND ULTIMATELY BRING ABOUT CONTROL OVER THE FLOW OF PRANA IN THE BODY.

CHANNELLING PRANA

Many ancient cultures, such as the Incas, Egyptians and Tibetans, believed in and taught breathing exercises for healing purposes and to raise consciousness. Mystics and gurus believed that practising pranayama led to the experiencing of the true self and the universe. The Christ talked about the sacredness of the breath in the Dead Sea Scrolls: 'We revere the holy breath which is beyond all creation. For behold, the eternal, highest realm of light, where the infinite stars reign, is the realm of air, which we inhale and exhale. And in the moments between inhalation and exhalation, all the mysteries of the eternal garden are hidden.' The Buddha used conscious breathing to achieve enlightenment and the Native American Indians and the Sufis include breathing practices in their initiation rites. The Indian guru Maharishi Mahesh Yogi, who developed the Transcendental Meditation technique, said: 'Through control of the breath we achieve control over the mind, and by controlling the mind we return to the original state of Eden.'

The ancient yogis measured a person's lifespan not in years but by the number of breaths they took per minute. They believed that a person who breathes in short, quick gasps is likely to have a shorter lifespan than a person who breathes deeply and slowly. This information they gleaned from animals living in the forest. They noticed that animals with a slow breathing rate, such as tortoises, elephants and snakes, lived longest, but animals with fast breathing rates, such as rabbits, birds and mice lived for a relatively short time.

The flow of prana
Pranayama shouldn't be seen merely as a set of breathing exercises that increase the body's intake of oxygen (although important), but also as a way to affect the flow of prana through the nadis, to purify them and induce physical and mental stability. The practice of kumbhaka (breath retention) brings about control of prana and eventual mastery of the mind – although this shouldn't be done until you've been practising yoga breathing regularly for some time. It's also important that when you start to retain the breath, either in or out, you apply these three bandhas or body locks.

Mula bandha – contraction of the perineum
Uddiyana bandha – pulling the abdomen under the rib cage
Jalandhara bandha – tucking the chin close to the chest to form the chin lock
Maha bandha – combining the three bandhas

Applying the bandhas unlocks and controls pranic energy, directing it into the 72,000 nadis present in the subtle body (one of the three bodies that make up human existence, together with the physical and causal bodies). From there, the energy can be directed into any part of the physical body to bring about balance. Ideally, you should learn the bandhas from a yoga teacher.

Yoga teaches that prana in the body is divided into five elementary parts, collectively known as the five pranas.

UDANA VAYU: Udana controls the parts of the body above the larynx. Thus the eyes, nose, ears and all sensory receptors are activated by this prana. Without it we'd be unable to think or be conscious of the outside world.

PRANA VAYU: This doesn't refer to the overall prana but to the part of the body in the region between the larynx and the top of the diaphragm. It's connected with the respiratory organs and the larynx, together with the muscles and nerves that activate them. It's the force by which we draw in breath.

SAMANA VAYU: Samana is connected with the region between the heart and the navel. It activates and controls the liver, intestines, pancreas and stomach. It also activates the heart and circulatory system, and is responsible for the assimilation of nutrients.

APANA VAYU Apana is responsible for the organs below the navel. It also influences the expulsion of prana through the mouth and the nose.

VYANA VAYU: This vital force pervades the whole body, regulating and controlling all movements of the body. It coordinates the other vital energies and activates the limbs, their associated muscles, ligaments, nerves and joints – and is also responsible for the erect posture of the body.

Prana is the medium that links the body with the soul. It's the connecting force between consciousness and matter, and it activates the physical body through the nadis. Primarily, pranayama ensures that the flow of prana throughout the etheric sheath (see page 33) is free and unimpeded so that the physical body is kept strong and healthy. For around 2 hours a day, either the right or left nostril is dominant. The flow of air through the left nostril is closely connected with the flow of prana in the pingala nadi, and the flow of air through the right nostril is linked with the ida nadi (see page 33). The only time when both nostrils are open is just before dawn, when the sushumna (see page 35) opens to allow the flow of the kundalini energy (see page 13). For this reason, meditation should be practised just before dawn.

BREATHING EXERCISES

Most of us breathe incorrectly, using only the upper part of our lungs. When our breathing is shallow, our body and brain can be starved of oxygen and life force. Shallow breathing also allows stagnant air to build up in the lower regions of the lungs. When you first start to practise deep breathing, it's important to listen to your body. Wear loose clothing so your body isn't restricted. Cotton clothing is preferable to synthetic fibres, which are believed to restrict the movement of our aura. Your spine should be in an upright position, with the shoulders taken back and down. This allows for expansion of the lungs and for the diaphragm to descend into the abdominal cavity during inhalation. If you start to become breathless, stop your deep breathing and return to normal breathing. If you start to feel dizzy, again stop your breathing exercise and return to normal breathing. Feeling dizzy could mean that you're hyperventilating or taking more oxygen into the body than it's used to.

Initially, practise your breathing exercises for a maximum of 5 minutes daily, gradually increasing this time as the body gets used to the greater intake of oxygen. Always practise in a well-ventilated room, preferably by an open window. And don't eat for at least 4 hours before practising asanas or pranayama. Try to stay focused on the breath throughout your practice time. Practising pranayama before working with the asanas that activate the triangles of light in the body is beneficial, because through the breath the nadis are recharged with pranic energy. If an exercise indicates retention of the breath, don't hold it for longer than is comfortable. For those who are new to pranayama, start with the first two exercises before moving on to the next, more advanced examples.

ABDOMINAL BREATHING

Lying flat on the floor, place one hand on your navel. Make sure that your chin is tucked in to prevent strain on the cervical part of your spine. If you find this difficult, place a small cushion beneath your head. When practising the exercise, make sure that you don't move your chest or shoulders. Inhale deeply, noticing how your hand rises with the expansion of your abdomen. Now deeply exhale and notice how the hand moves down as your abdomen contracts. Continue to practise for around 5 minutes.

CHEST BREATHING

Lying on the floor with your arms by your side and your chin tucked in, inhale and expand your chest while keeping the abdominal muscles contracted. Notice how the whole of your rib cage starts to expand, moving outwards and upwards. Exhaling, notice how the rib cage collapses as the ribs move inwards and downwards. Try not to move the abdomen during this exercise.

YOGA COMPLETE BREATH

This exercise combines the two exercises above. With practice, it allows the optimum amount of air to be taken into the lungs and the maximum amount to be expelled. The exercise can be practised sitting on a straight-backed chair, with both feet on the floor and the hands placed palms-down on the thighs, or sitting on the floor in either the full or half lotus posture, if you're already familiar with these, or with the legs stretched out in front of the body – again with the hands resting palms-down on the thighs.

First, exhale fully through the nose. Now start your slow, smooth inhalation, expanding first the abdomen and then the chest until the maximum amount of air has been taken into the lungs. Now exhale by releasing air first from the chest, then from the abdomen and finally by contracting the abdominal muscles to allow the maximum amount of air to be expelled from the lungs. The inhalation and exhalation should take the same length of time, so when you first practise this exercise you might find it helpful to count to seven for both the inhalation and exhalation. If the count of seven is too long for you, reduce the count to four or five. If the count is too short, then increase the number to a count that feels comfortable. With practice, you'll find that you're able to increase the count on both the inhalation and exhalation.

ALTERNATE-NOSTRIL BREATHING

The breathing technique sukh purvak, or alternate-nostril breathing, maintains a balance in the constant interplay of positive-negative pranic currents. Everywhere in the external world, we encounter manifestations of the positive-negative principle. We find it in the composition of the atom, in the cell, in the polarity of the Earth, in the sun and moon, and in the man and woman relationship. In those dimensions of existence that we gradually come to perceive through our inner vision, the same negative-positive relationship occurs.

Sitting either on a chair or on the floor, make sure that your spine is straight and your body relaxed.

1 Place your right thumb lightly against your right nostril, your index and middle fingers on your forehead, between and just above your eyebrows, and your fourth and little finger lightly against your left nostril (see opposite).
2 Exhale deeply through both nostrils.
3 Press the left nostril closed with your fourth and little fingers and quietly inhale deeply through the right nostril to a count of eight.
4 Close both nostrils and retain the breath for a count of four, applying the three bandhas (see page 56).
5 Release the bandhas, open the left nostril and exhale through it to a count of eight.
6 Close both nostrils, apply the bandhas and hold the exhalation to a count of four.
7 Release the bandhas and inhale through the left nostril to a count of eight.
8 Close both nostrils, apply the bandhas and retain the breath for a count of four.
9 Release the bandhas, open the right nostril and exhale through it to a count of eight.
10 Close both nostrils, apply the bandhas and hold the exhalation to a count of four.
11 Release the bandhas and inhale through your right nostril to a count of eight.

This completes one round. Without pausing, perform ten more rounds – increasing the number of rounds with practice. Your aim is to eventually breathe in to eight, hold for eight, breathe out to eight and then hold the breath out to a count of eight. When you first work with the exercise, it's advisable to omit retaining the breath. Retention of the breath, with the application of the bandhas, can be practised at a later date. On completion of this exercise, place your hands on your thighs and breathe normally for a few minutes.

Alternate-nostril breathing is an indispensable prelude to meditation. It brings about calmness and tranquillity and clears the nadis. The flow of prana in the ida and pingala nadis is equalized, and the whole body is nourished by the extra supply of oxygen. This leads to an improvement in your health.

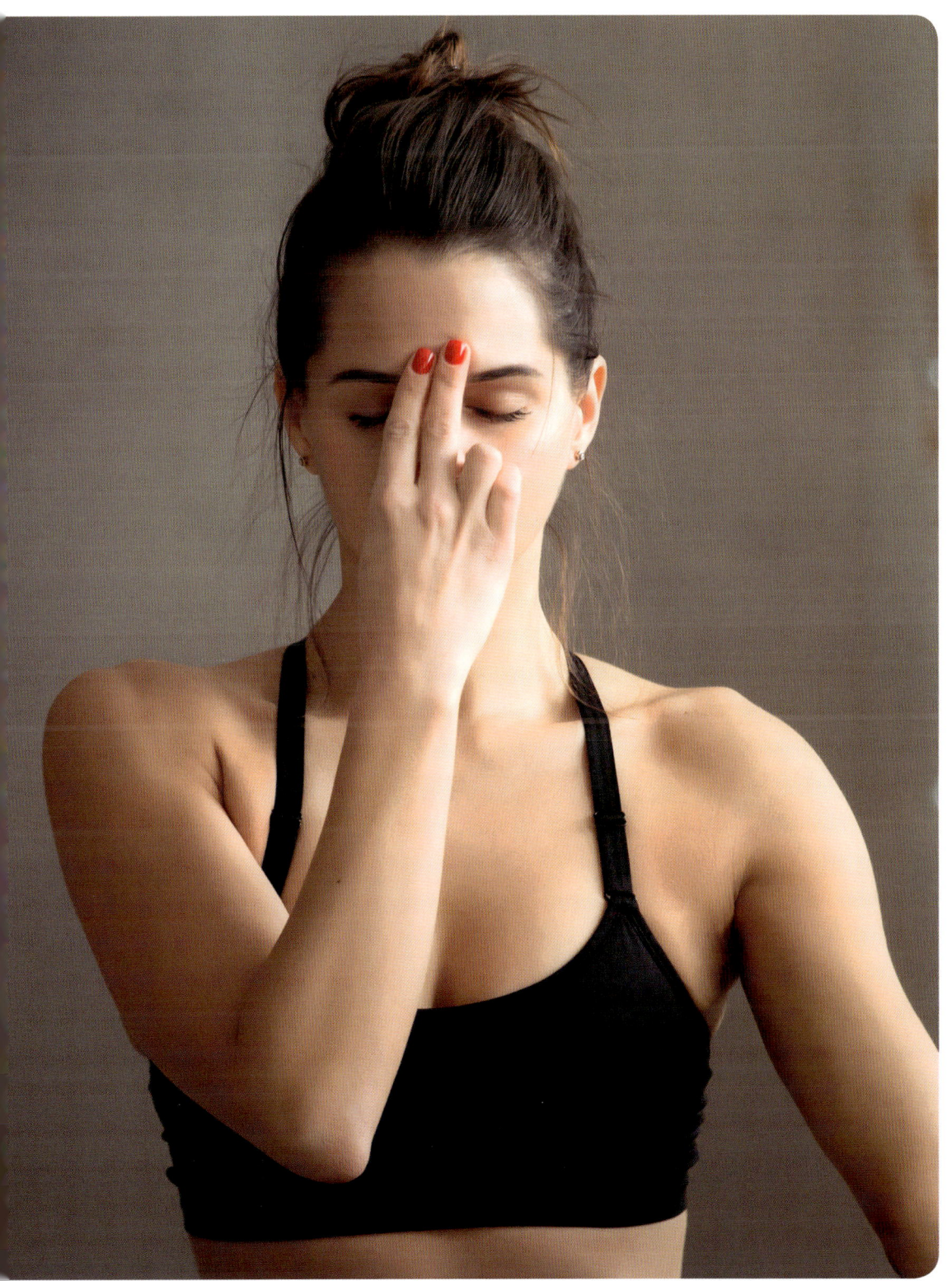

VISUALIZING WHITE PRANIC LIGHT

When you've become familiar with the alternate nostril breath, bring into it the visualization of white pranic energy. During each inhalation, visualize breathing in an intense white light. Imagine the light circulating throughout all the nadis in order to cleanse and vitalize them. When you exhale, visualize breathing out any disharmony.

Humming breath

Sit either on a chair or on the floor, and make sure that your spine is straight and your body relaxed. Breathe in deeply. Then, on a slow exhalation, hum softly to make the sound of murmuring bees. Continue for as long as is comfortable.

This breathing exercise is helpful prior to relaxation and for those who suffer from insomnia. When you've finished, lie down on the floor and relax.

Cooling breath

Sit either on a chair or on the floor, and make sure your spine is straight and your body relaxed. Place your hands on your thighs. Form your mouth into an O shape. If you can, fold the sides of your tongue to form a narrow tube and extend this just outside the mouth. Inhale slowly and deeply through the folded tongue. Relax the mouth and exhale slowly through your nose. Start with nine rounds and, over time, gradually increase this to sixty rounds. Because the tongue is a mirror image of the whole body, inhaling air through the folded tongue cools the air we're inhaling, thereby cooling the whole body.

This breathing exercise initiates relaxation and tranquillity of mind. It also encourages a free flow of prana throughout the body.

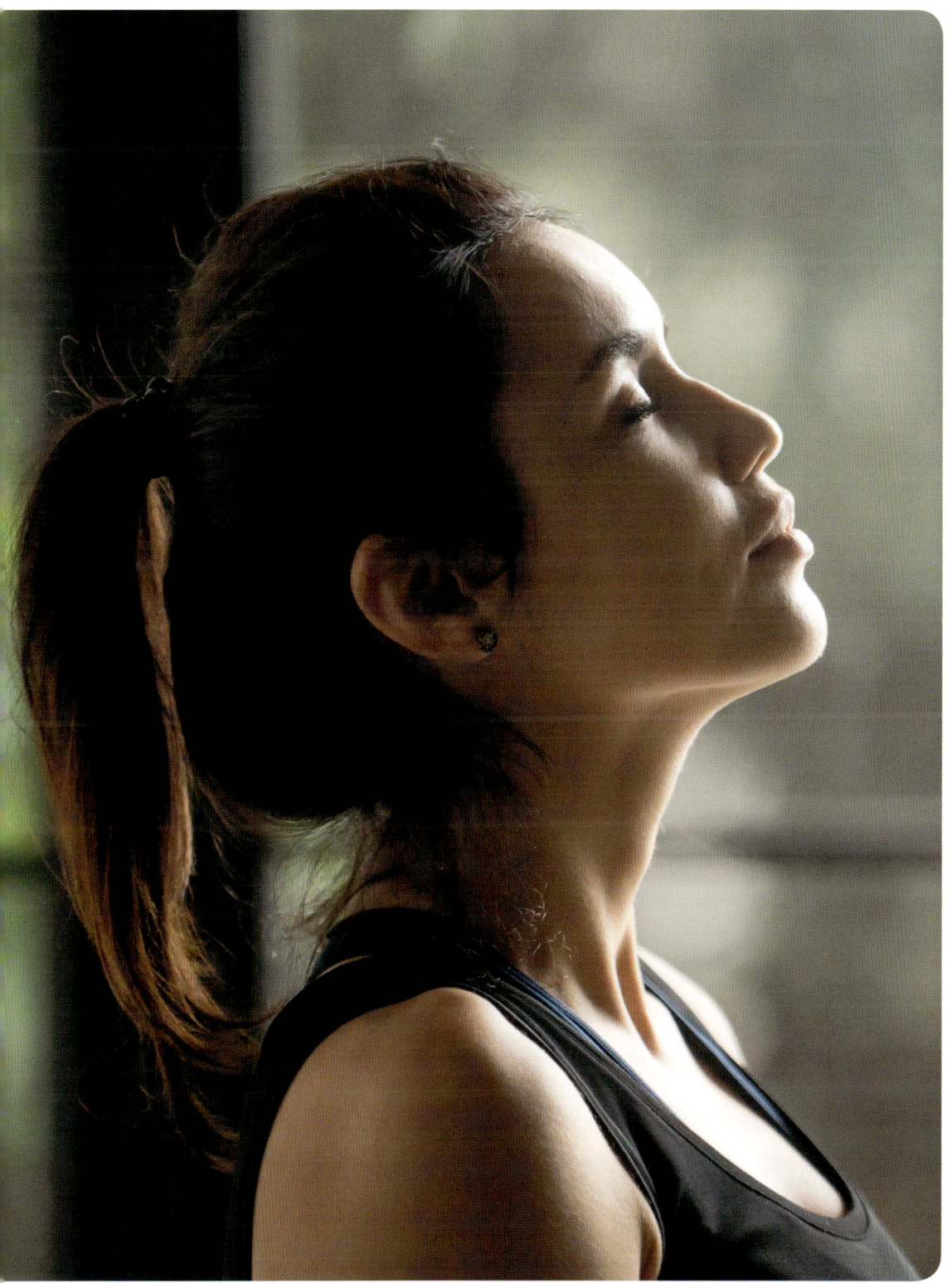

VILOMA PRANAYAMA

This breathing exercise involves a series of interrupted inhalations or exhalations with pauses, hence its name: 'viloma' means 'against the grain', or 'against the natural order'. The exercise can be performed either in a sitting or lying position. If you're sitting, keep the back erect and the head lowered, so the chin rests in the notch between the two collar bones.

Version 1 (interrupted inhalation) is especially beneficial for those with low blood pressure. If you suffer from high blood pressure, follow version 2 (interrupted exhalation); it's also recommended that you perform the exercise lying down.

Caution: Don't perform this exercise if you have heart problems.

Version 1

1 When you're ready to begin, inhale for 2 seconds then pause for 2 seconds; holding the breath, again inhale for 2 seconds and again pause for 2 seconds, holding the breath. Continue in this way until the lungs are completely full.
2 Now hold the breath in for 5–10 seconds.
3 Now exhale slowly, making a humming sound as in the humming breath (see page 62).
4 This completes one cycle. Repeat for ten to fifteen cycles.

Version 2

1 With the chin resting in the notch of the neck, take a deep breath through clenched teeth to a hissing sound.
2 When the lungs are full, hold the breath for 10–15 seconds.
3 Now exhale for 2 seconds, then pause for 2 seconds; exhale for 2 seconds three pause for 2 seconds. Continue in this way until you've expelled as much air as possible from the lungs.
4 This completes one cycle. Repeat a further ten to fifteen times, then lie down and relax.

It's recommended that you master the humming breath before working with this breathing exercise.

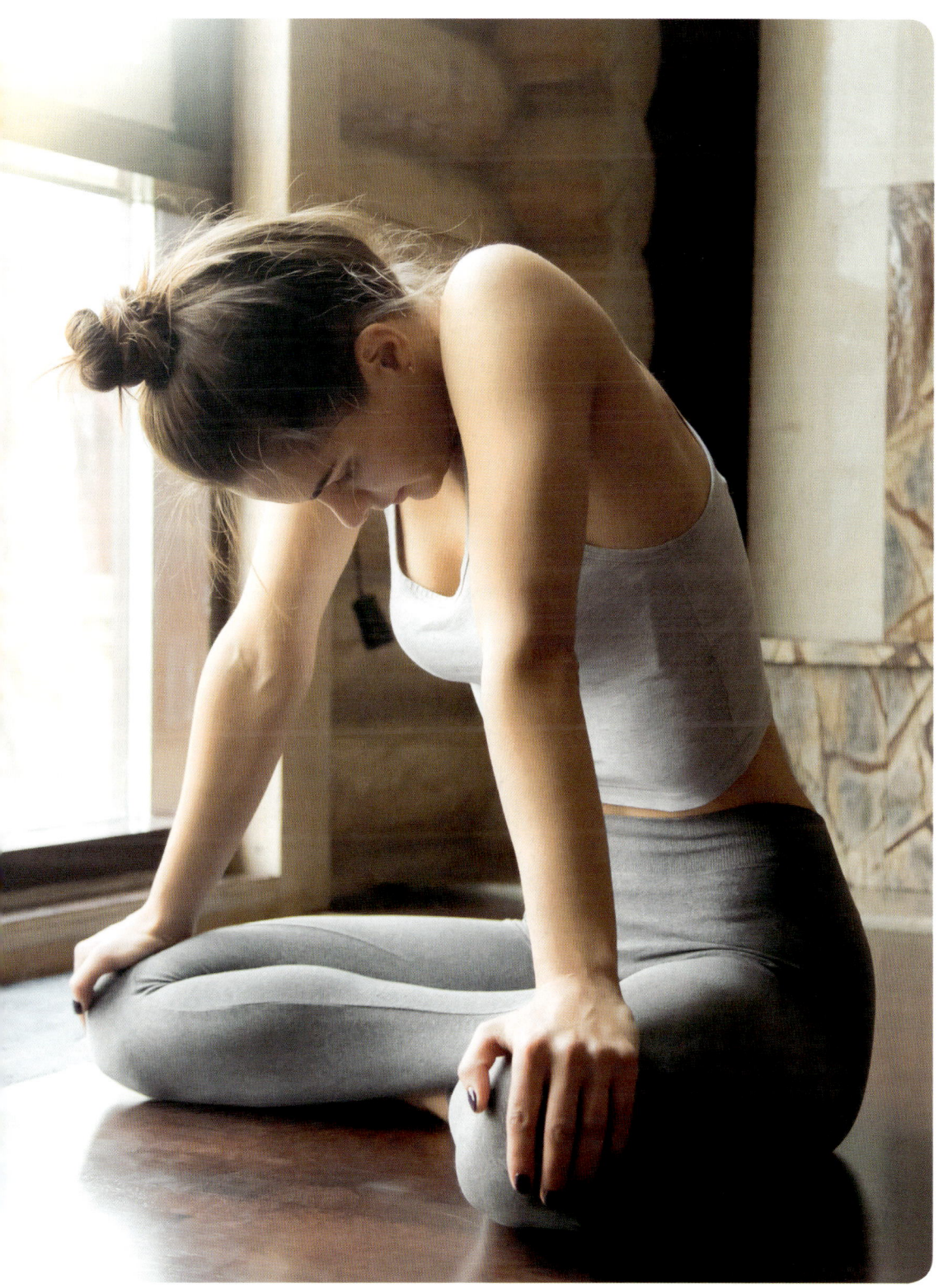

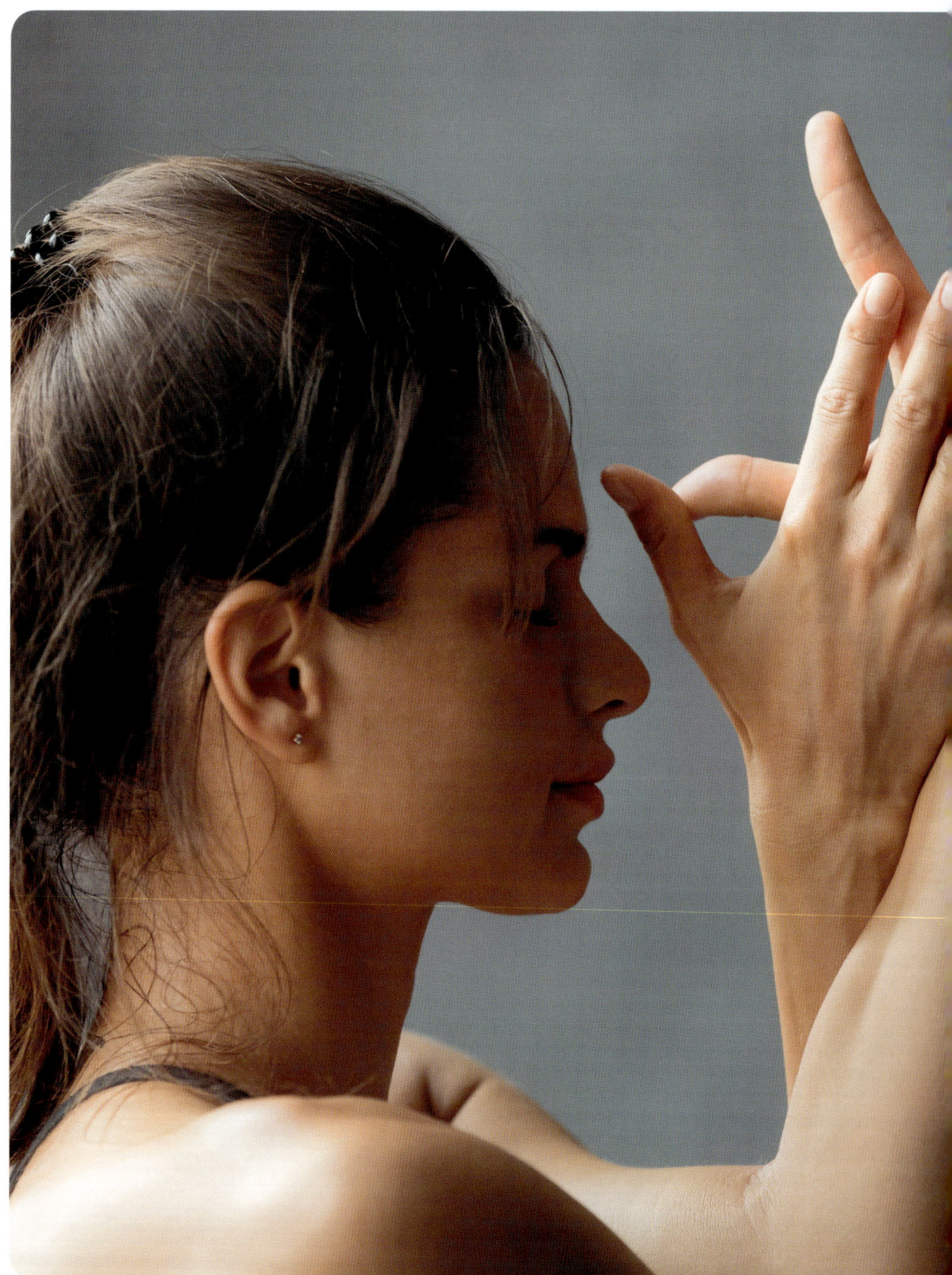

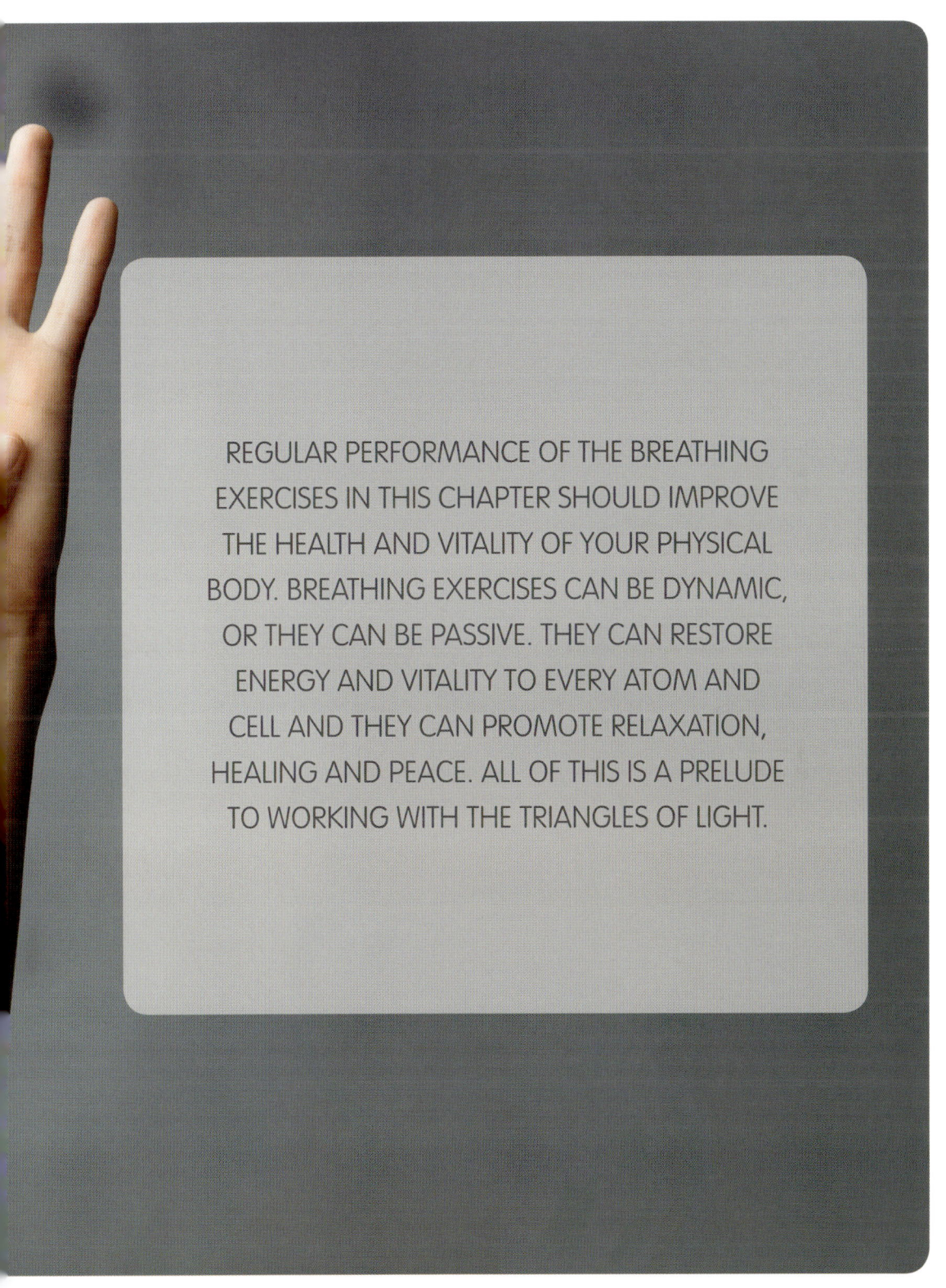

REGULAR PERFORMANCE OF THE BREATHING
EXERCISES IN THIS CHAPTER SHOULD IMPROVE
THE HEALTH AND VITALITY OF YOUR PHYSICAL
BODY. BREATHING EXERCISES CAN BE DYNAMIC,
OR THEY CAN BE PASSIVE. THEY CAN RESTORE
ENERGY AND VITALITY TO EVERY ATOM AND
CELL AND THEY CAN PROMOTE RELAXATION,
HEALING AND PEACE. ALL OF THIS IS A PRELUDE
TO WORKING WITH THE TRIANGLES OF LIGHT.

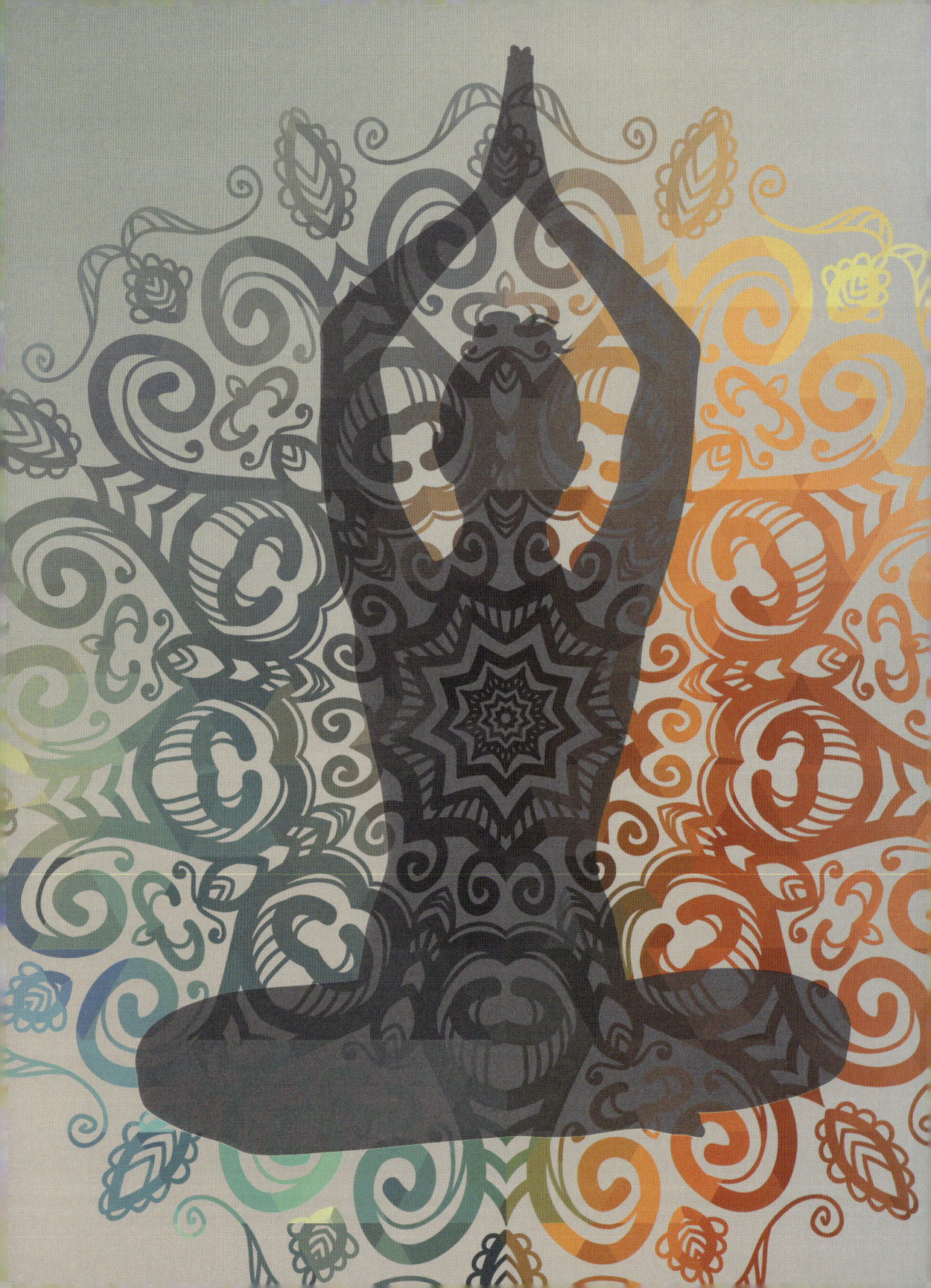

5

WORKING WITH THE CHAKRAS

TO EXPERIENCE THE TRIANGLES OF LIGHT FORMED
IN CERTAIN YOGA POSTURES, IT'S IMPORTANT
THAT YOU BEGIN TO FAMILIARIZE YOURSELF WITH
THE CHAKRAS THAT ARE INSTRUMENTAL
IN FORMING THOSE TRIANGLES.

CHAKRA PREPARATION

The following simple exercises, visualizations and meditations will help you to become familiar with the chakras. The exercises provide a gentle introduction for anyone whose body isn't very supple – and they also act as warming-up movements for the classical asanas of yoga that form the triangles of light.

Food and drink

When practising yoga, you should not have eaten for at least 4 hours. The first law of yoga is non-violence, and this applies to your physical body as much as to anything else. Practising yoga on a full stomach interferes with the digestive process, which isn't beneficial to your body. You can, however, drink as much water as you need.

The right routine

Practise in a room that's warm, quiet and well ventilated, and where you'll not be disturbed. Ideally you should have a non-slip mat, a foam block and a reasonably long belt for your practice. These can be acquired from any shop selling yoga accessories.

If, at the start, you find it difficult to hold a posture, don't be disheartened. Each of us has to work with the stage we're at, and with regular practice we become more proficient. Try to practise at the same time each day. This forms a good habit and ensures that your yoga session becomes part of your daily routine. Wear loose, comfortable clothing, and preferably start and end each session with a period of relaxation. A relaxed body moves more easily into postures than a tense one does. When practising, you can work through all the exercises in this chapter, in the order they're given, or, if your time is limited, you can take on one or two chakras each day. You might also like to record your progress in a diary. I'm sure that once you start to experience the benefits of yoga, you'll want to practise it every day.

Those of you who are already conversant with yoga and able to maintain the asanas forming the triangles of light, will, as you work with these on a regular basis, notice very subtle changes taking place at a physical, emotional, mental and spiritual level.

EXERCISES TO START
YOUR PRACTICE SESSION

Stand either against a wall or in the middle of the floor. Your feet should be slightly apart and parallel, with the toes on each foot aligned. Make sure that your spine is straight. For this exercise, imagine that your spine is the trunk of a tree and that all the nerves radiating from your spinal cord are the tree's branches.

Breathing in, raise your arms above your head and form a cup with your hands (see right). Gently close your eyes and visualize a beam of brilliant white light pouring from the soul star chakra into your cupped hands. From your hands, it flows down into the top of your head and into the crown chakra. This warm, brilliant, soft white light then flows down your spine – the trunk of your tree – and into all the nerves that form the tree's branches. As your inner tree becomes flooded with light, visualize it energizing and revitalizing all your body cells and all the organs and muscles served by your nervous system. When your body has become filled with this energizing light, on an exhalation lower your arms down to your sides. If you wish, you may repeat this exercise until your body feels energized and vibrant.

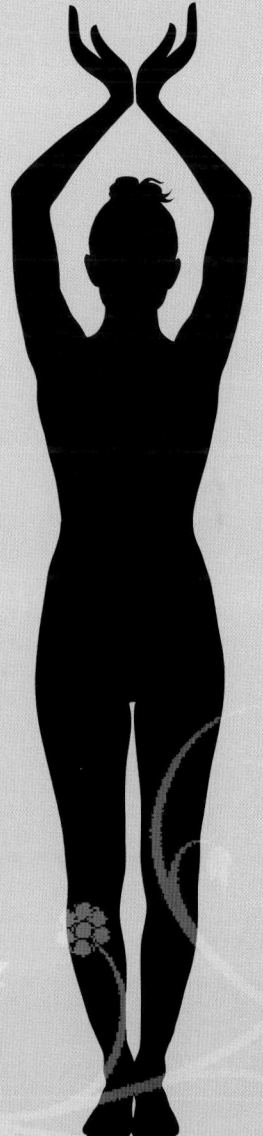

BASE CHAKRA

Sit on the floor, with your back against a wall and a cushion placed in the small of your back. Press the soles of your feet together and draw them as close to the body as possible (see below). Then place the palms of your hands on your thighs and gently start to lower your knees towards the floor. When you've lowered them as far as possible, bring your concentration into the base chakra, visualizing this as a brilliant, clear red orb of light.

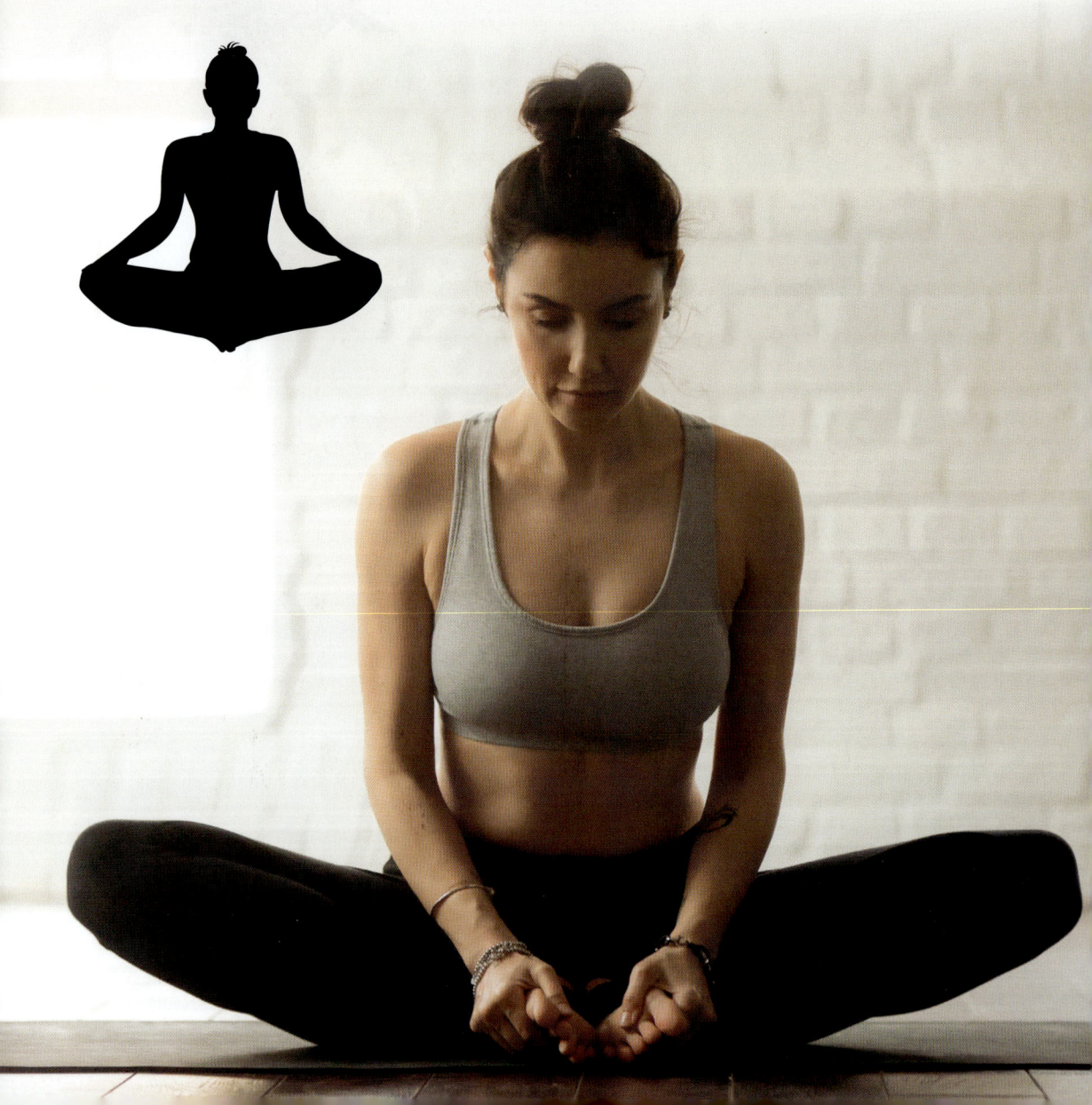

An alternative posture is to sit on the floor, with your legs stretched out in front and the spine straight. Bend your knees, placing the soles of your feet by your buttocks. Your feet should be approximately 15 cm (6 in) apart. Take your arms between your legs and under your knees. Exhale, and recline the trunk slightly backwards to raise the feet from the floor and allow you to balance on your buttocks (see right). Your spine should be kept straight throughout. Hold the posture for as long as is comfortable. Keep your concentration on the base chakra, visualizing it as an orb of brilliant, clear red light.

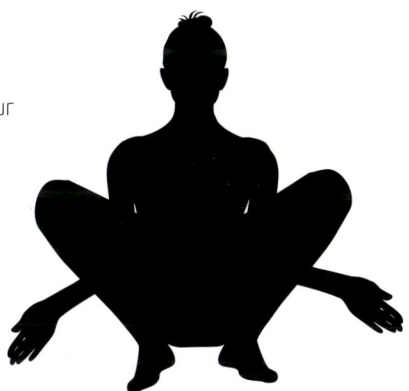

VISUALIZATION WITH THE BASE CHAKRA

When you've completed either or both of the above exercises, sit either on the floor or on a chair, making sure that the spine is kept straight. If you're sitting on a chair, place both your feet on the ground.

Visualize yourself standing barefoot in the garden. Imagine that you have roots coming from the soles of your feet and going deep down into the earth, giving you a firm anchor. Now bring your concentration to the base of your spine – the coccyx, where the base chakra is situated. This chakra forms the first rung of our ladder, the place where we begin our spiritual journey. It's our incarnating chakra, the centre that places our feet firmly on the ground. Visualize the centre as a pulsating orb of clear red light. With each exhalation, imagine a beam of light travelling from the base chakra down both legs and into the roots extending from your feet into the earth. Try to feel the warmth and energy this colour gives to the base of your spine and your legs, and the sense of security that the firm base – the earth that you're standing on – is creating for you. If we don't create a firm base on which to build our spiritual life, it's easy to stumble and fall. If your concentration starts to wander, gently bring it back to the task in hand.

When you feel ready, gently open your eyes and feel any changes that may have occurred within you.

SACRAL CHAKRA

For this posture, if you find it difficult to bend forwards from your hips, you'll need either a foam block or a large book to sit on. This helps to project the body forwards from the hips. If you can't touch your feet with your hands, you may also need a belt.

Sit either on the floor or on your block or book, with your legs extended in front of you. Inhaling, straighten your spine and take your hands down to your feet. (If you can't touch your feet, place a belt around them, holding it at either end.) Keeping the spine straight and the knees locked, exhale, and slowly lower the trunk of the body as far down onto your legs as you can (see below). This posture works with the hamstring muscles, so if these aren't supple you may be unable at first to lower your body very far, although, with regular practice, it will become much easier. While holding the posture, bring your concentration into the sacral chakra, just below the navel, visualizing it as a bright orange orb of light. When you're ready, inhale and come slowly back to the sitting posture.

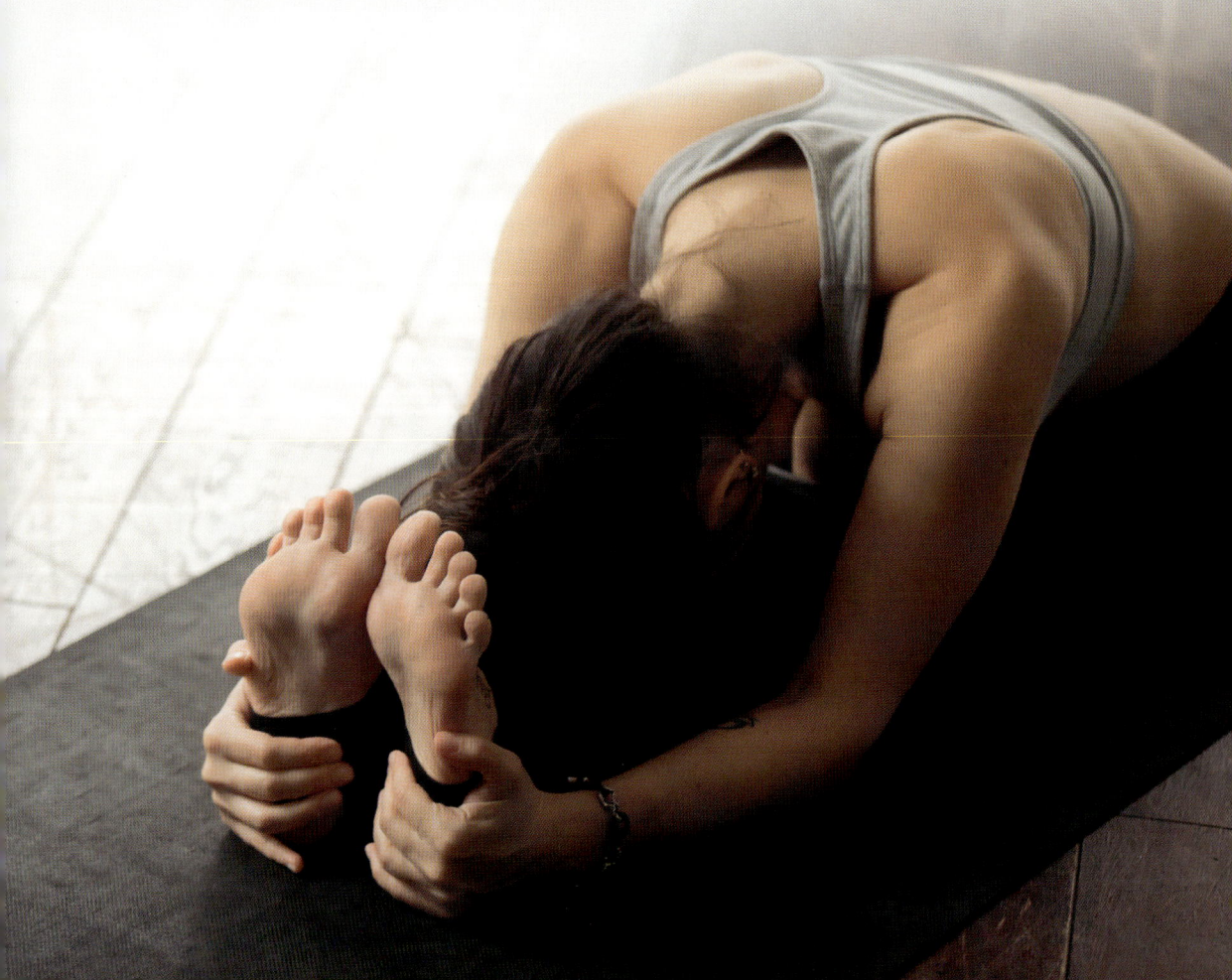

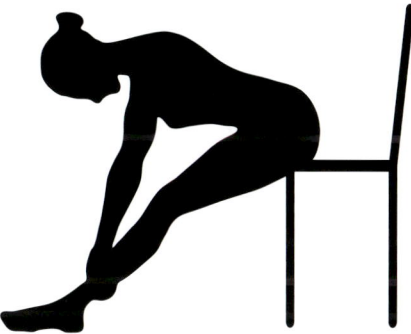

If your body is very stiff, you can practise this posture from a chair. Sitting on the edge of your chair, with your legs extended in front of you, place your hands on your thighs and slowly slide your hands down your legs as far as you can (see right). When you've reached this point, concentrate on the sacral chakra as described opposite.

VISUALIZATION WITH THE SACRAL CHAKRA

The sacral chakra is connected with feminine energy and the water element. When women work with this chakra they need to review their lives to find whether or not they're honouring and nurturing themselves. More generally, this chakra challenges us to flow freely through life – if we lack that flow we must look to ways of removing whatever is obstructing it.

Imagine that you're sitting on the bank of a gently flowing brook on a warm summer's day. Lying on the bed of the river are stones and boulders of various sizes, the larger of these jutting out of the water. Notice how the river smoothly winds its way around these stones and boulders as it happily wends its way to its outlet, the sea. Now visualize what would happen if these stones and boulders piled up against each other. The water would build against the stones until the dam they had formed was eventually broken by the force of the water. Now imagine the rocks and boulders as your unresolved emotional issues and the water as the tears shed as emotions are released. If you let your emotional issues remain unresolved, your life force, wanting to flow freely through the nadis, will eventually try to break down the blockages you've created. Failing this, the only outlet for these emotional blockages is through the physical body, resulting in physical disease.

As you reflect on this scene, consider whether any barriers or problems in your own life are restricting your life force's flow, preventing you from evolving as a spiritual being. Having looked at any such restrictions, consider ways of resolving them.

Before ending this exercise, visualize an orb of clear, bright orange light radiating from your sacral centre, and allow this colour to flood your body with energy and joy.

SOLAR PLEXUS CHAKRA

This movement can be done sitting either on the floor or on a straight-backed chair. If you're working from a chair, sit sideways on the chair, with both feet placed on the floor. Turn from your waist so your chest is facing towards the back of the chair (see below left). When you've turned as far as you can, bring your concentration into your solar plexus chakra, visualizing it as a golden sun whose rays of warm light penetrate all parts of your body. Hold the posture for as long as is comfortable, then take your legs to the other side of the chair and repeat the movement with the opposite side of your body.

If you're sitting on the floor, sit sideways, with your legs either outstretched alongside a wall or bend the knee nearest to the wall and place the foot on the outside of the outstretched leg (see below right). From your waist, slowly turn towards the wall, trying to place your whole chest against it. Place your hands on the wall, on either side of your chest. While holding the posture, visualize the golden sun radiating from the solar plexus chakra. Repeat on the opposite side.

After completing the above movement (it can be repeated several times), sit comfortably on your chair or on the floor and use the following visualization.

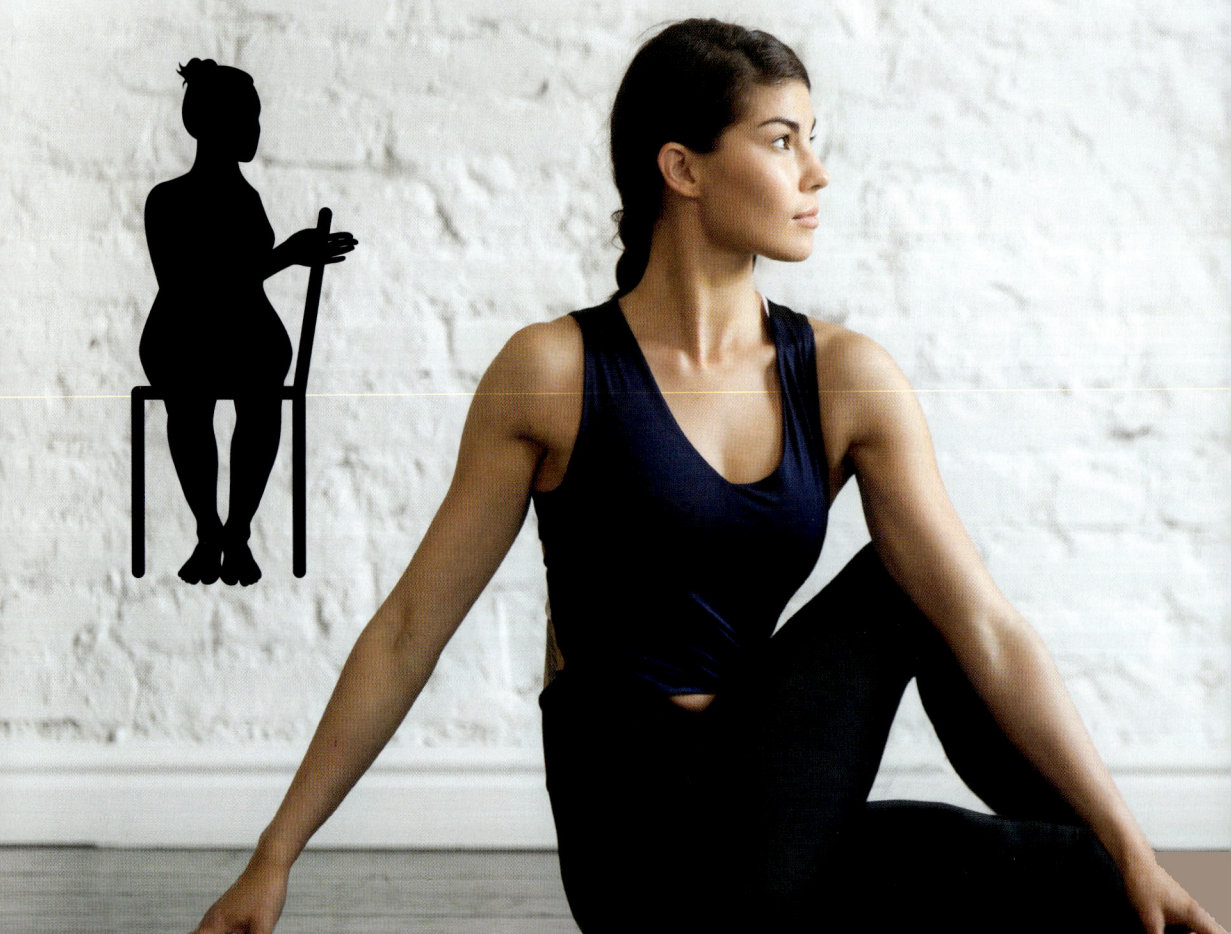

VISUALIZATION WITH THE SOLAR PLEXUS CHAKRA

The solar plexus chakra is where our fears and emotional upsets are stored, a centre connected to the sun and the element of fire. It's also the centre where heat is produced through digestion, a process that can be disturbed by emotional turmoil.

Imagine that you're sitting on a deserted beach on a warm summer's day. As the sun's rays play on your body, they help you to relax and be at peace. The only sounds you hear are the rolling of waves across the golden sands and the cry of seagulls.

Bring your concentration into your solar plexus chakra and imagine that a large golden sun resides there, creating a warm glow in and around this part of your body. The sun is vital to life – without it everything on our planet would die. We're beings of light and need the pranic light energy from the sun to energize and nourish us. The sun symbolizes the supreme Cosmic Power present in every human, the eternal part of us that came from the Supreme Being, the part we're striving to remember. When we do start to remember, tremendous changes take place in our life. We're able to see the good in all things and we have a new zest for living. Eventually, we attain the state of enlightenment where we become one with God.

Visualize the golden yellow of the sun and feel its warmth detach you from everyday problems, from fears and worries and from friends and family. In this state, you can understand that the actions of those around you are part of *their* learning process and should be blessed, not judged. Golden yellow is the colour that helps us to achieve the wisdom and insight we need to make the right life choices. A bright golden yellow can give us courage, whereas a dull, dirty yellow is the colour of cowardice.

Remembering that this solar plexus centre is where our fears and emotions are stored, quietly consider any such turmoil in your own life. Fear is one of the most destructive emotions. It casts a grey shadow that prevents us from finding our inner light, and also from working with the chakras situated above the solar plexus. Try to recognize the cause of your fears and emotional disturbances, and ask your higher self for the wisdom to resolve them. As you recognize your fears, express each one verbally. Actually voicing our fears and worries helps to balance the solar plexus centre. As you do this, visualize the rays from your solar plexus sun dispersing any negative energy surrounding you. If you begin to lack courage, feeling that you can't attempt what you know to be the right solution for you, reconnect to your golden yellow sun, envisaging it at your solar plexus, glowing with an ever brighter, clearer colour as you express each fear and worry.

Whenever you experience emotional turmoil or fear in your life, immediately connect to your solar plexus's comforting golden sun.

HEART CHAKRA

Sitting either on the floor or sideways on a straight-backed chair, make sure that your spine is straight and that your shoulders are drawn down and back. Place your hands by your sides, and gently rotate the shoulders in a clockwise direction. All the work should come from your shoulders, leaving your arms and hands being completely relaxed. Feel the gentle release of any tension in your shoulder muscles. Now rotate your shoulders in an anticlockwise direction. Work with this exercise for 1–2 minutes. Next, take your hands behind your back and clasp your fingers, making sure that your hands are at right angles to your wrists (see right). This position helps to activate the energy centres at each wrist.

Take your shoulders back to open your chest, and gently raise your arms. Don't bend your back or lean forwards to try to raise your arms higher – this won't achieve anything. Hold the position initially for a count of five then, on an out-breath, slowly lower your arms. Still maintaining the hand and arm position behind your back, rest for a count of five, then repeat the movement. This time, while holding the posture for as long as is comfortable, bring your concentration into your heart chakra, visualizing it as a pale pink lotus flower sitting on a bed of spring green leaves. When your arms tire, relax them and place your hands on your thighs. Follow this movement with the visualization given below.

VISUALIZATION ON THE HEART CHAKRA

Sit comfortably, with a straight spine and with your shoulders drawn down and back so your chest is open. Start by breathing in and out to a count of five to enable you to quieten your mind and become focused.

Now bring your concentration to your heart chakra, which is situated slightly to the right of your physical heart. Visualize this as an orb of green pulsating light. As you concentrate on this centre, it starts to expand until it completely surrounds you, with you sitting at its centre – the centre of what could be described as a circular room. The floor of this room is carpeted in white and filled with a pale, ethereal green light. At the room's centre is a large, open pale pink rose. The edges of its petals are varying shades of pink – from the deepest, almost red pink to the very palest pink.

A lighted candle stands at the centre of the rose. A gentle breeze blows through the room, making the flame dance and twist into many shapes and sizes, sometimes sending minute sparks of brilliant light into the surrounding atmosphere. Looking into the flame, you see an equal-limbed cross of light, which reminds you that the heart centre is our centre of balance. Looking at the vertical line of the cross reminds us of our duality: the left and right sides of our body; the left and right hemispheres of the brain; our creativity and intellect. To become whole, we need to work at integrating our opposites. Looking at the horizontal bar of the cross reminds us that the three chakras above the heart chakra are connected to our spirituality, and the three lower chakras – which we have already worked with – are linked to our physical life. The flame of the candle represents the light of our divine self, while the air element stands for the challenges that life presents us. If the flame is weak, it could be extinguished by the softest of breezes; but if the flame is strong, then even a mighty gale will only make it glow more brightly.

Shift your gaze from the flame to the rose. The various shades of pink correspond to earthly, physical love – but as we move into the rose's pale pink centre, that earthly love changes into unconditional love.

Reflecting on all of this, consider how you're coping with life's challenges. Are they making you a stronger person, or are you collapsing under their weight? What are your thoughts on unconditional love – a love free of judgement? Is this hard for you? Do you find yourself constantly criticizing and judging your friends and acquaintances? If so, what measures should you take to change this? This reminds me of a passage I read on the life of Pope John Paul II. What stood out clearly was the fact that he visited, in prison, the man who tried to assassinate him, and gave that man total forgiveness.

As you reflect on the heart chakra, you may feel that in order to become more aware of your spiritual self and a more whole and balanced being, you're being challenged to change things in your life, however hard that may be. Spend a little time dwelling on these thoughts before ending this visualization.

Concentrate on your heart chakra, visualizing it as an orb of green pulsating light.

THROAT AND ALTA MAJOR CHAKRAS

The following simple exercise will help to relax your neck muscles and make them supple. Some of yoga's classical asanas use these muscles, but they're also important when you work with the throat and alta major chakras. If you have neck problems, or have at any time experienced whiplash, work very gently with these movements.

Sit either on the floor or on a straight-backed chair, and place your hands on your thighs. Your back must be kept straight and your shoulders down and relaxed throughout these movements. It's easy to raise the shoulders or bend the back to move further into the posture – but doing so achieves nothing. Try to remain conscious of this while you hold each movement for a count of five, slowly increasing to a count of ten.

On an in-breath, and keeping your teeth together and your mouth closed, gently tilt your head backwards as far as you can. Feel the muscles along the front of your neck being stretched and freed from tension. Breathing out, raise your head, and on the next out-breath bend your head forwards to stretch and release any tension in the muscles at the back of your neck. Breathing in, raise your head and, on the next out-breath, take your head over towards your left shoulder, stretching the muscles along the right side of the neck. Breathing in, raise your head and, on the next out-breath, take your head over towards your right shoulder to stretch and release tension in the muscles along the left side of your neck. Repeat this series of movements as many times as you like.

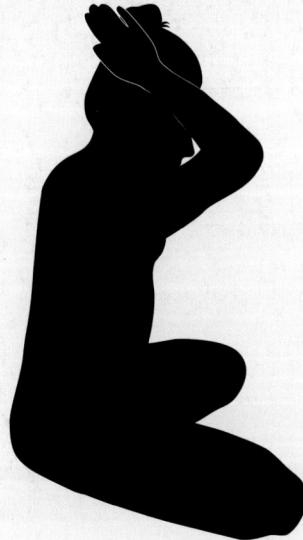

Now, clasping your fingers, place your hands on the back of your head (see left). Gently press your head forwards until your chin rests between the two clavicle bones. This position is known as the chin lock and is instrumental in working with the throat and alta major chakras. Initially, you may find the chin lock difficult, but daily practice with the above neck movements will make your neck muscles supple and allow you gradually to achieve the position.

With your head lowered as far as possible, through the gentle pressure of your hands, focus on the alta major chakra, which is situated at the medulla oblongata – roughly at the base of the skull. Visualize a stream of white pranic energy flooding this centre and flowing to all parts of your physical body to supply it with the energy it needs to maintain optimum health. Hold this position and concentrate on the visualization for as long as possible. If your mind wanders, gently bring it back to the task in hand.

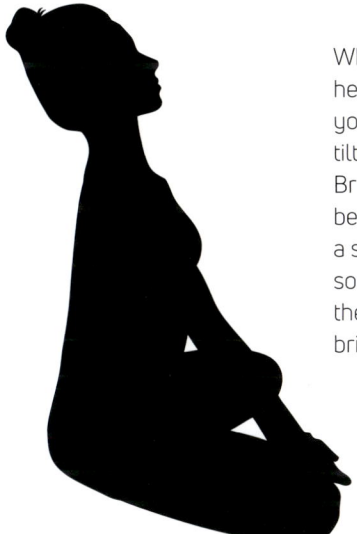

When you're ready, on the next in-breath raise your head, lower your hands onto your thighs and, keeping your teeth together and your mouth closed, gently tilt your head backwards as far as you can (see left). Bring your concentration to your throat chakra, situated between the two clavicle bones. Visualize this centre as a sky blue lotus flower, made vibrant by a beam of clear, soft blue light descending into your crown chakra and then into your throat. Visualize this lotus flower becoming brighter and more lustrous.

On the next in-breath, raise your head. Clasp your fingers and place them again on the back of your head (see right). Gently press the head down until your chin rests between your two clavicle bones. Now visualize a narrow beam of bright white light coming from the alta major chakra to join with the throat chakra. Hold this visualization for as long as is comfortable, then, on an in-breath, raise your head and sit for a few minutes reflecting on your experience.

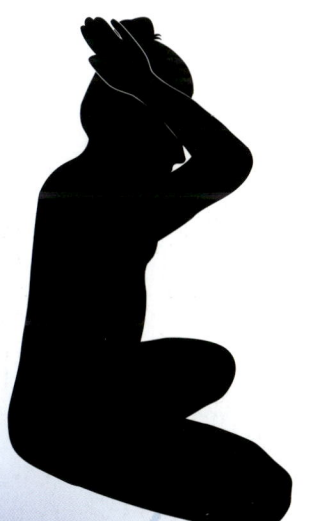

This was the first line of light
I experienced. Over many months,
I discovered that this beam of white light
played a major role in the formation
of the light triangles.

BROW CHAKRA

Sit either on a straight-backed chair or on the floor. With the index finger of your right hand, massage, in a clockwise direction, your brow chakra, located between your eyebrows (see below). Continue to do this for 2–3 minutes. Now place both hands on your thighs. Close your eyes and raise them to look up into the brow chakra. (At first, your eyes may become very tired after only a few seconds, but with daily practice they'll become stronger and able to hold this position for any length of time.) Practising this eye position is important because the closed eyes focus on the brow chakra during meditation and also when working with some of the classical asanas instrumental in forming the light triangles. Remember that the brow chakra is the door through which we enter higher states of consciousness.

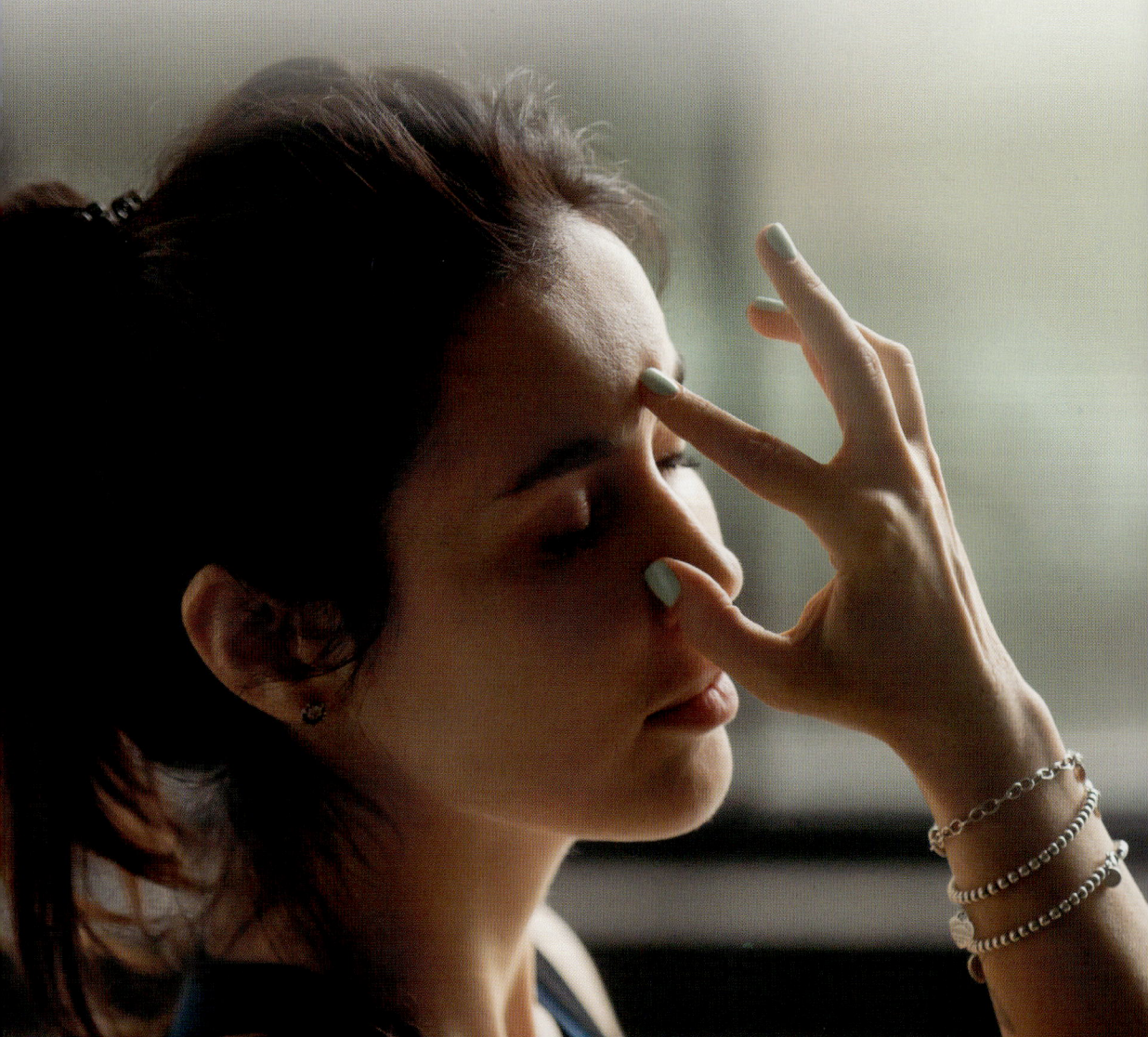

MEDITATION ON THE BROW CHAKRA

Sitting in your chosen place, with your concentration focused on the brow chakra, visualize it expanding to encompass you in a sea of indigo light – the colour of a cloudless night sky. Feel and breathe in the silence and stillness of this infinite space, the void from which all became manifest. In the stillness, contemplate who you really are. Most people identify themselves with the physical body and the name given it at birth, but what happens when our physical body wears out, dies and returns to the elements from which it was originally made?

Think about the idea of God or the Supreme Being, present at the beginning of time and needing to experience its supremacy. To do this, the Supreme Being had to send forth a vibration through which it could manifest the various aspects of itself in different forms. One of the forms it assumed was mankind. When it had incarnated into our human form, it made us forget who we really are and gave us freedom of choice by allowing us free will. Through this gift of choice, we come to appreciate and realize our divinity. We're able to appreciate what is good by experiencing the bad; our understanding of joy comes from our encounter with sorrow; our comprehension of light stems from knowing the darkness. The knowledge and acknowledgement of this duality enables us to begin the process of bringing that duality back to wholeness. When we finally achieve this, the brow chakra fully opens and we experience the joy and bliss of recognizing our true self. The aim of all spiritual paths, including the path of yoga, is to regain the knowledge that we are God made manifest, and co-creators with It. We can be shown ways of achieving this, but, ultimately, each of us has to find our own way back to our eternal home.

To end this meditation, visualize your brow chakra resuming its normal size, and reconnect with your physical body by gently increasing your inhalation and exhalation. Then slowly open your eyes.

When you focus on this chakra, visualize it as a bowl of deep indigo light. Gaze into the indigo light and imagine a six-pointed star of light at its centre. The brilliance of this star draws you gently to it and, eventually, encompasses you in a wonderful feeling of peace and ecstatic joy.

Bringing your focus back to the indigo light, visualize the colour flooding around your body, giving you a deep sense of peace and relaxation.

Gaze into the indigo
light and imagine a six-pointed
star of light at its centre.

CROWN CHAKRA

Either stand upright, or sit on a straight-backed chair with both feet placed on the floor. Raise your arms over your head and form a cup with your hands. Now bend your elbows to allow the heel of your hands to rest on the crown of your head (see below). Take your elbows as far back as possible. Visualize a beam of white cosmic energy flowing from the soul star chakra – the centre that collects cosmic energy – into the cup formed by your two hands. As the energy enters your hands it turns from white into a soft pale violet light, which then pours down into your crown chakra. Envisage the chakra as a purple lotus flower still in bud. As the violet light pours into and envelops this flower, it opens, and each petal becomes alive with a clear, shimmering violet light. When the flower is bathed in violet light, it helps to restore balance to your pineal gland and all the other elements that constitute your brain.

 When you're ready, lower your arms to your side (see right), or, if you're sitting on a chair, place them palm upwards on your lap. Still concentrating on your crown chakra, try to feel the energy pulsating from this centre.

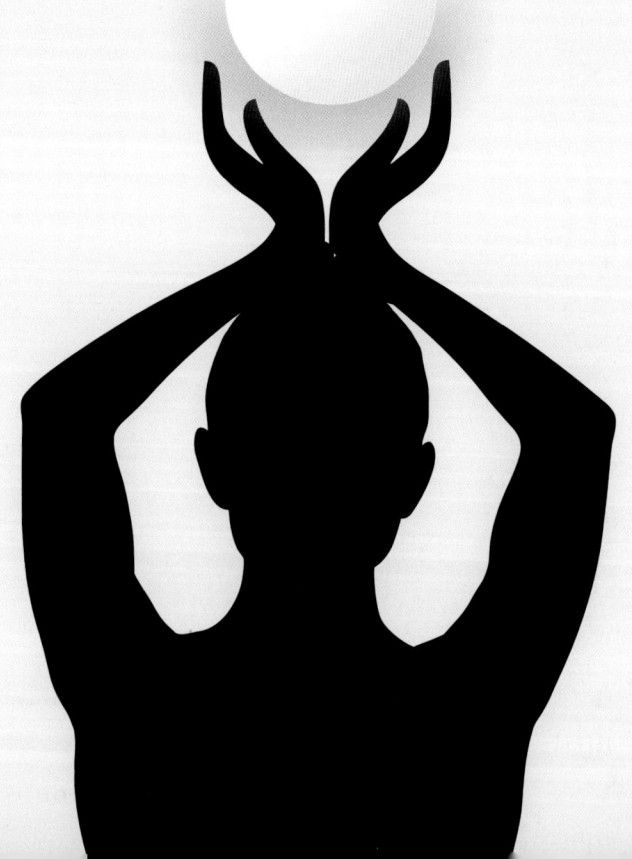

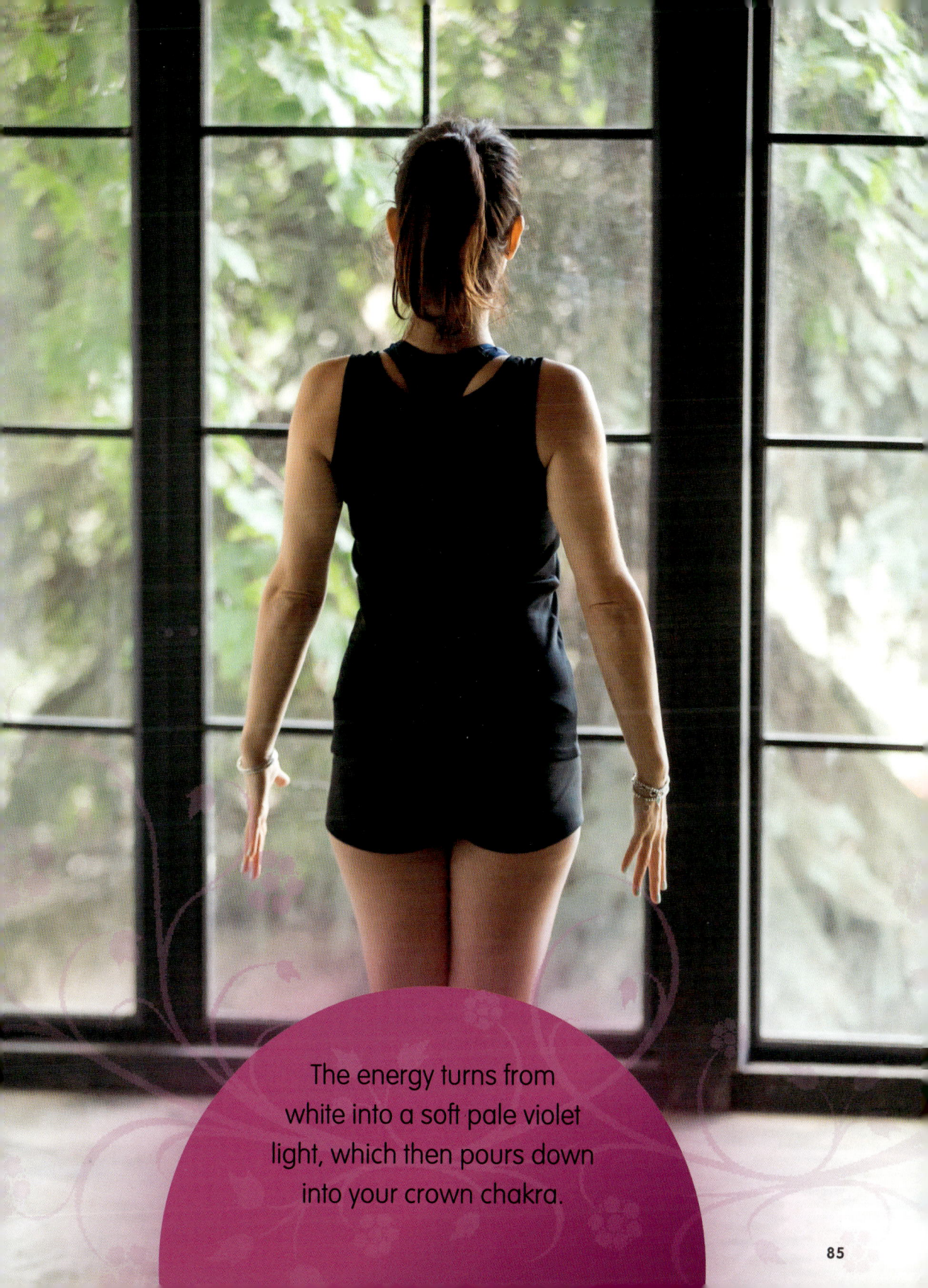

The energy turns from
white into a soft pale violet
light, which then pours down
into your crown chakra.

SOUL STAR AND EARTH CHAKRAS

Stand with your back and heels against a wall. Stretch your arms over your head, keeping them straight, and join the palms of both hands. Bending your left knee, place the sole of the left foot against your inner thigh (see below). Keeping both buttocks on the wall, gently move the bent leg as far back to the wall as you can manage. It's important not to twist from the waist to achieve this. While holding this posture, visualize a beam of white light coming from the soul star chakra, through your hands into the crown chakra, and then flowing down into the heart chakra. Next visualize a beam of red light coming from the earth chakra, through your right foot, up through the three lower chakras and then into the heart chakra, where it merges with the white light. Here, the two beams of light turn into a very pale pink light – the colour of unconditional love – which vibrates throughout the heart chakra. Hold this posture for as long as is comfortable before changing over legs and repeating on the opposite side.

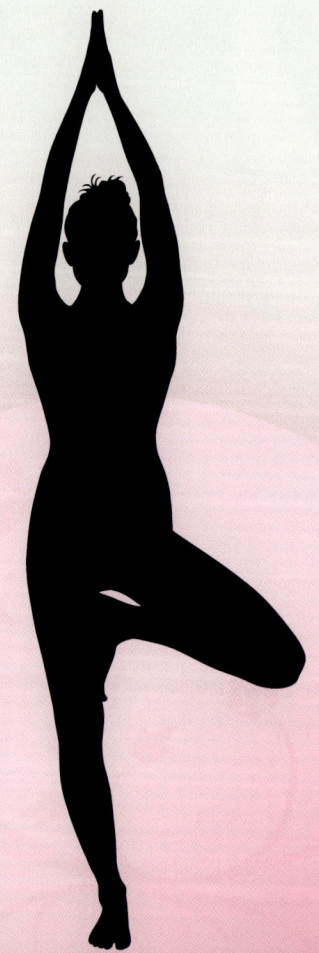

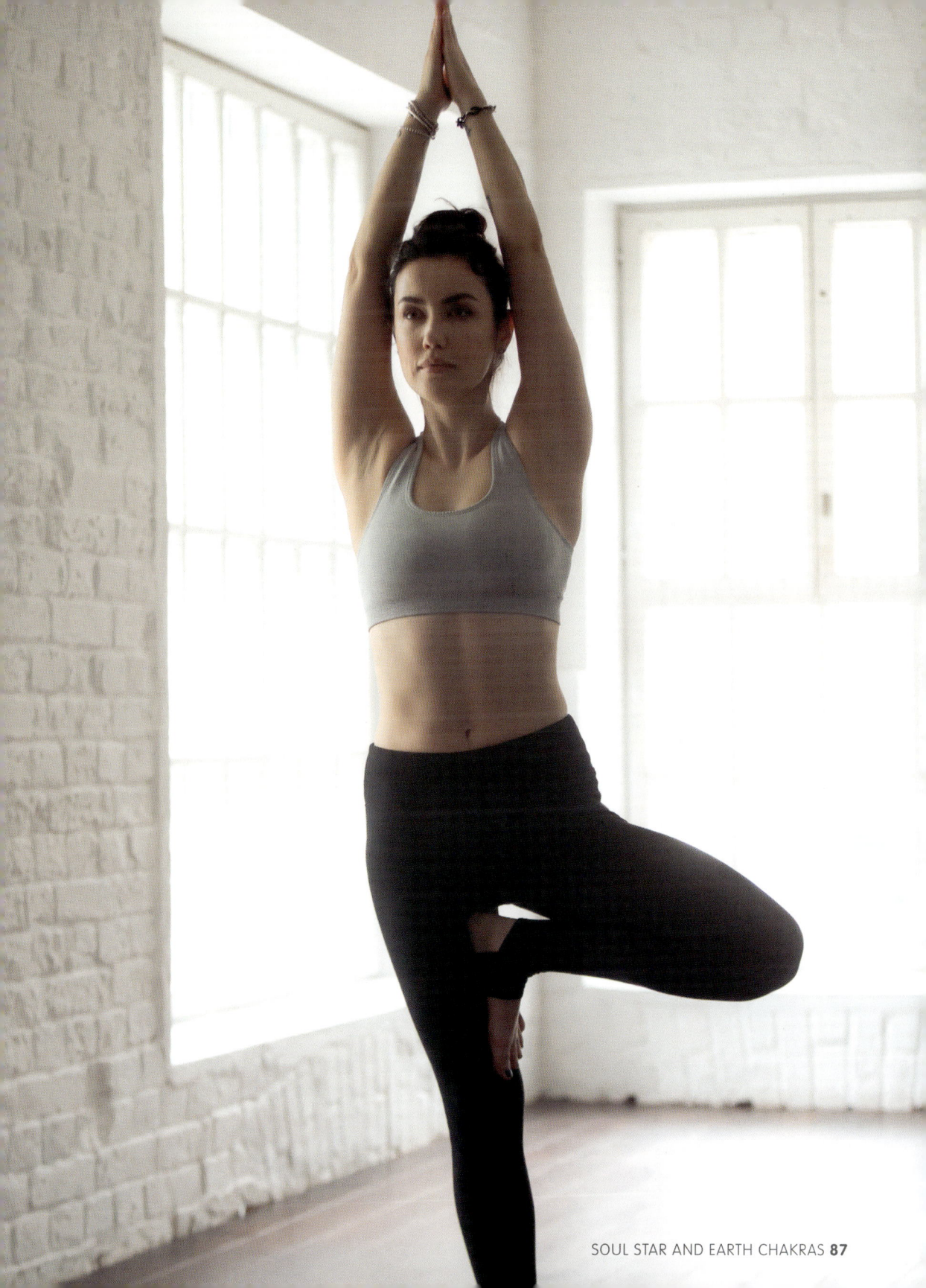

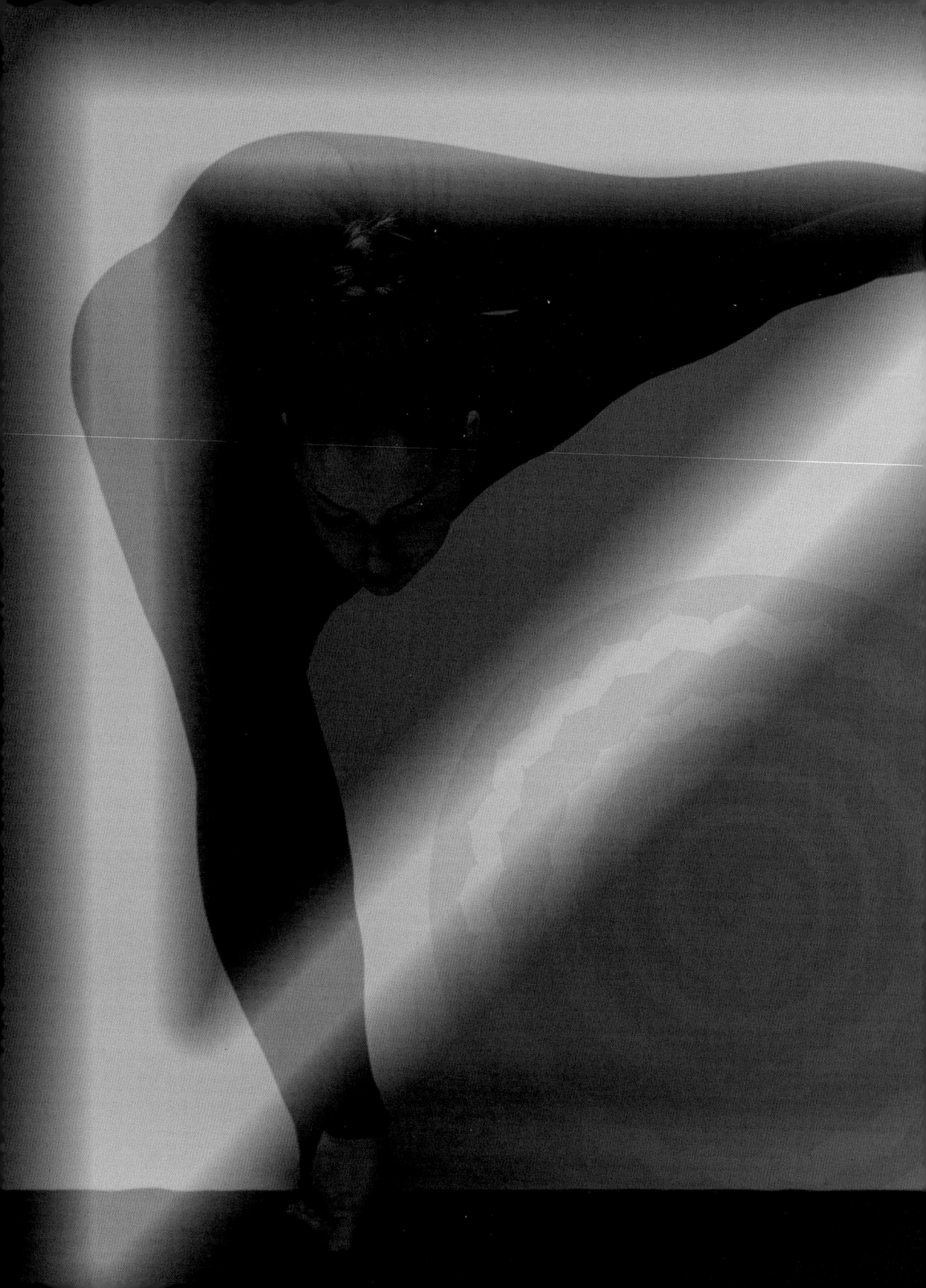

6

THE TRIANGLES OF LIGHT

AS YOU ENGAGE THE ENERGY LINES THAT FORM
THE TRIANGLES OF LIGHT, YOU WILL DISCOVER
HOW VISUALIZING – AND, EVENTUALLY, FEELING
– THESE TRIANGLES AS YOU PRACTISE THE
POSTURES ENERGIZES THE BODY, ALLOWING YOU
TO CONNECT TO OUR OWN INNER LIGHT.

USING THE TRIANGLES

With each of the following asanas, more than one triangle of light is formed. First practise your chosen asana, holding it for as long as is comfortable, then repeat it to work with the triangles of light. At first, visualize just one of the asana's triangles. Then each time you work with this asana, you can visualize a different triangle of light. When you feel ready, you can start to visualize all of the triangles.

When you've formed the triangle or triangles present in the asana you're practising, visualize them filling with white pranic light, energizing and bringing into balance the parts of the body each triangle works with. At first you may have difficulty visualizing the triangles, but with practice it becomes much easier. Remember, we're beings of light and we need light for our well-being.

A new dimension

At this time in Earth's history, the planet and its inhabitants are on the verge of a quantum leap into the fifth dimension. We're already starting to move from the third dimension, one very much connected to our emotions, our thoughts and our earthly survival, into the fourth dimension – one where we have to look at ourselves and let go of everything that we no longer resonate with. It's a dimension where all institutions are breaking down in order to facilitate new growth and a new way of living. This isn't a very comfortable period, but one that's necessary if we and all things on Earth are to move into the fifth dimension.

One of the key issues we have to contend with is fear. This emotion has the power to stop us moving forwards into the light of our true being. Endeavouring to overcome fear and other negative emotions and thoughts will enable us to pass eventually through the fourth into the fifth dimension. Another challenge when we pass through the fourth dimension is to start working to open the heart chakra – the chakra of unconditional love.

One way to open the heart chakra is to visualize any triangle involving that chakra filling with pale pink light. Pink is the colour of unconditional love.

Energy of light

Before starting to work with the triangles of light, practise this energizing relaxation technique. Lie on the floor, making sure your body is straight. Then extend both your arms horizontally, with your palms facing upwards. Keep your legs together and tuck in your chin to ensure there's no undue pressure on your cervical spine. Then spend a few moments relaxing your body.

When you're ready, visualize a triangle of light forming between the minor chakra on the palm of each hand and the earth chakra, situated approximately 15–20 cm (6–8 in) below your feet. Now visualize a second triangle, formed by the minor chakra on the palm of each hand and the solar star chakra, situated approximately 15 cm (6 in) above the crown of your head.

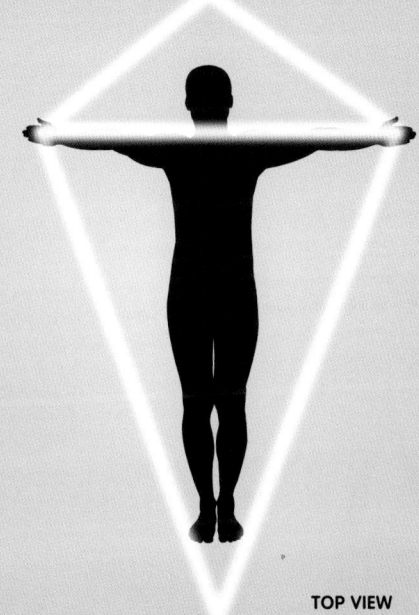

TOP VIEW

As you inhale, visualize a beam of white light coming from the soul star chakra, down through the crown chakra and into the upper triangle. Continue to bring this light down until the upper triangle is filled with light. Using the same technique, bring the light down into the lower triangle. When this triangle is filled with light, you'll find yourself lying in a two-dimensional octahedron of white light. The octahedron is related both to the element of air and to the heart chakra. Try to feel the light that fills the octahedron, energizing and revitalizing every atom and cell in your body. Working with this exercise will gradually enable you to feel the minor chakras in the hands and feet as a warm, pulsating heat, which gradually extends into every part of your body. Continue to work with this for as long as you feel comfortable.

NAMASKAR (salutation posture)

Sit comfortably in a cross-legged position. If this is difficult for you, sit on a cushion. As you inhale, stretch your arms up over your head, bringing the palms of your hands together. Look up towards your hands.

This posture opens the chest, lifts up the spine and helps the knee and hip joints. It's good preparation for some of yoga's classic asanas.

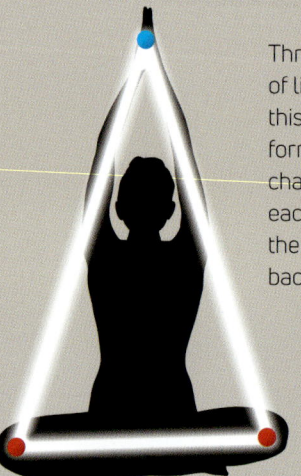

Three main triangles of light are created in this posture. The first is formed with the minor chakra on the palm of each hand and with the minor chakra at the back of each knee.

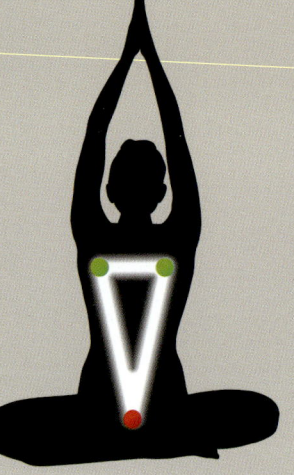

The second triangle is formed with a minor chakra behind the nipple of each breast and with the base chakra.

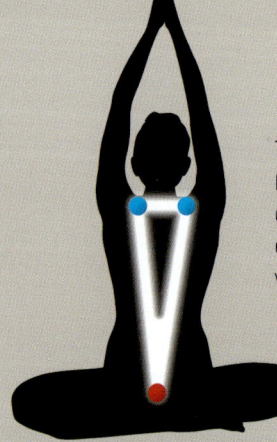

The third triangle is formed with a minor chakra halfway along each clavicle bone and with the base chakra.

While you hold the posture, either concentrate on one of the triangles or try to visualize all three. Each time you practise this posture, you may choose to work with a different triangle.

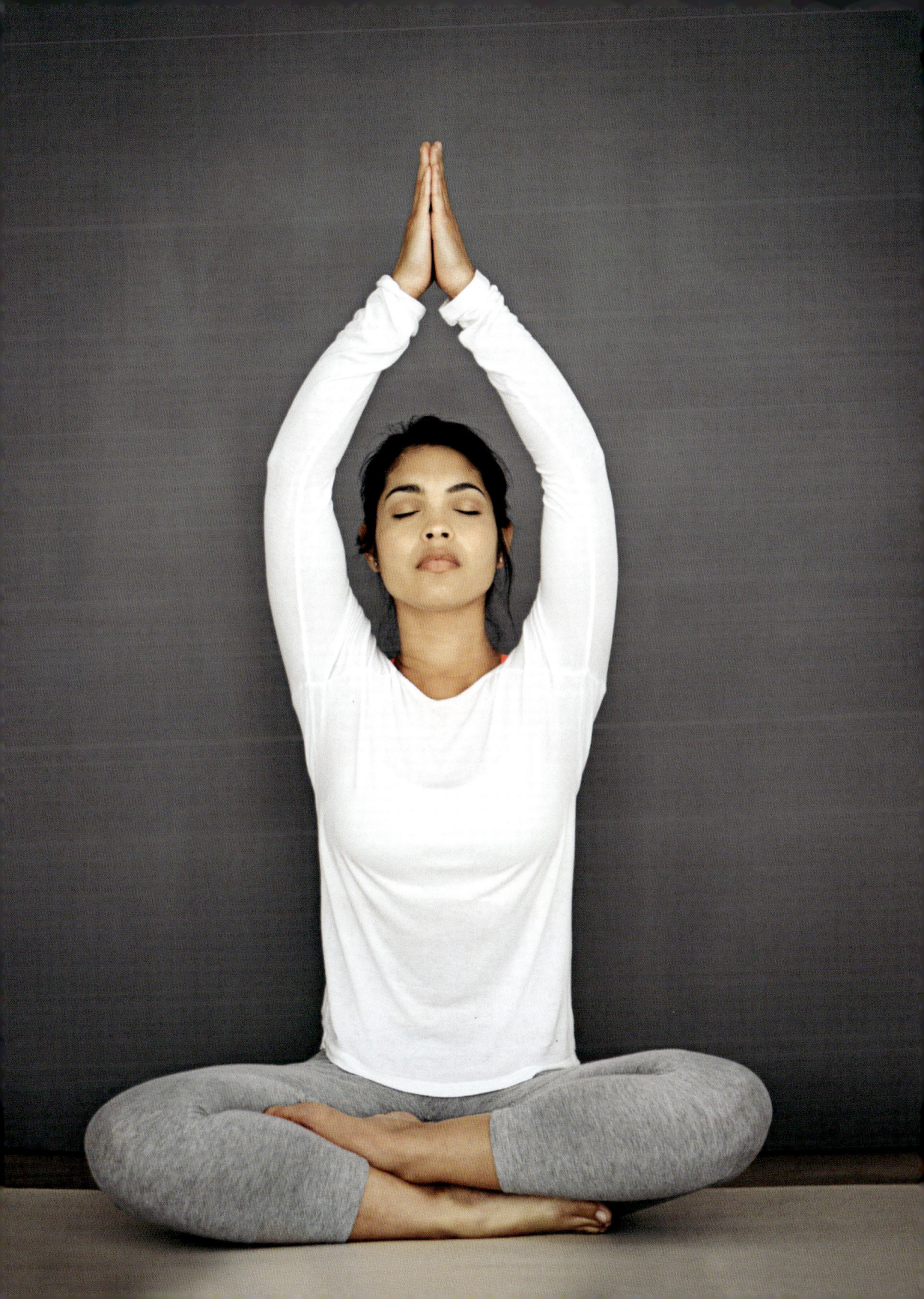

YOGA MUDRASANA (psychic union posture)

Sit in either full lotus, half lotus or simple cross-legged posture. Make sure that your spine is straight. Inhaling, clasp your hands behind your back. Exhaling, keeping your spine straight, move your trunk forwards from the hips until your forehead (or chin, if you're able) touches the floor. At the same time, raise your arms upwards (see opposite). If at first you're unable to go fully into the posture, move your trunk forwards as far as you can – but taking care not to bend your spine. If you can't touch the floor with your head, rest it on either a folded blanket or a book.

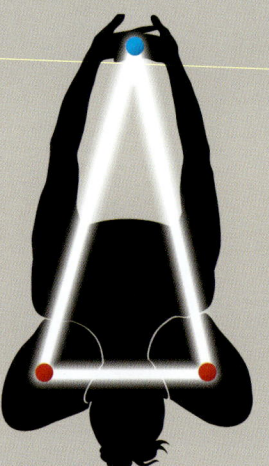

Two triangles of light are formed in this posture. The first is with the minor chakra on the palm of each hand and with the minor chakra behind each knee.

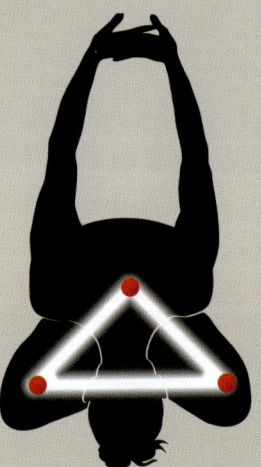

The second triangle is formed with the base chakra and the minor chakra behind each knee.

This posture, which works primarily with the base chakra, relieves stiffness in the arms and shoulders. It also improves digestion and relieves constipation by intensifying contraction and relaxation in the intestines.

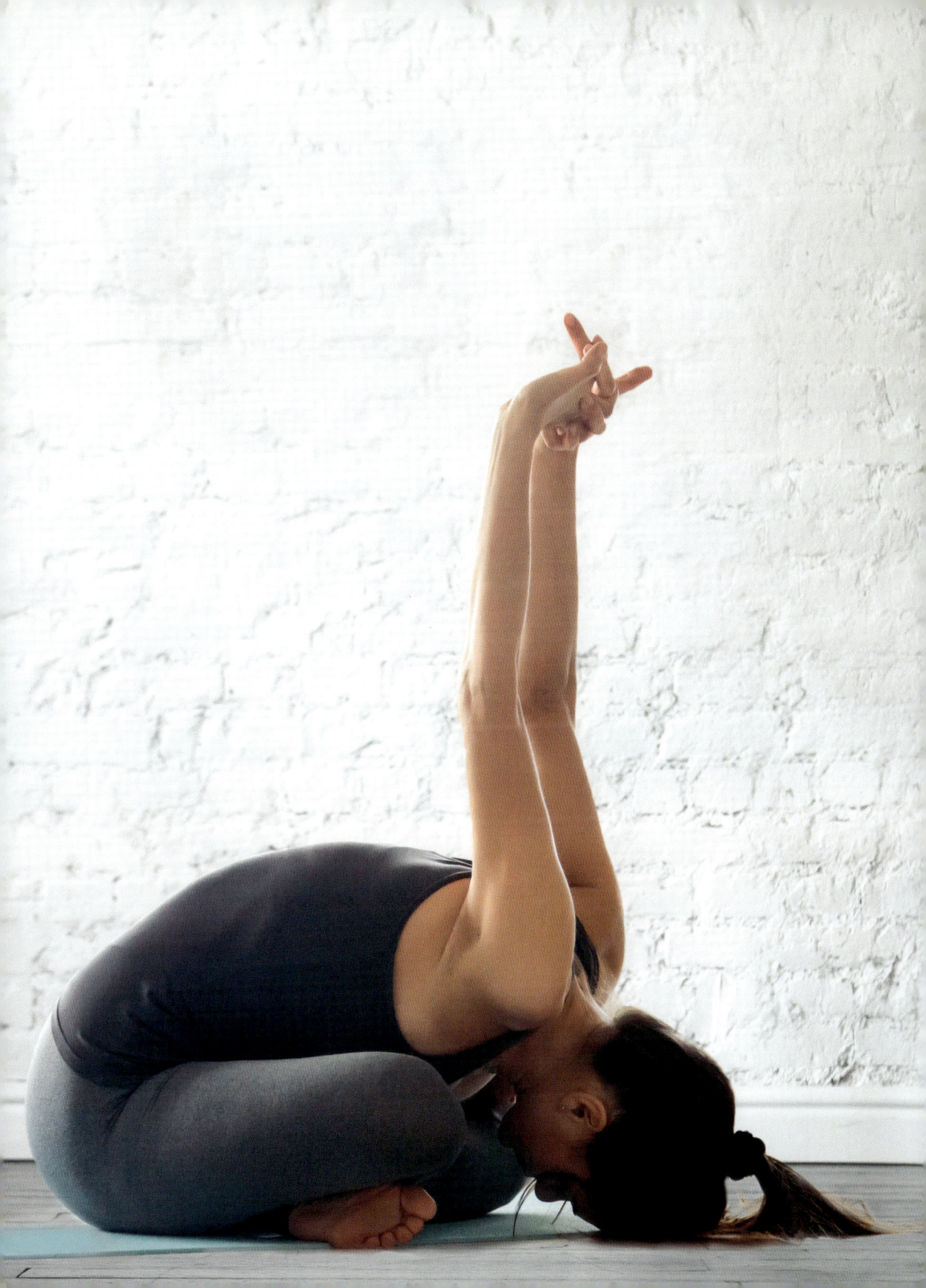

JANU SIRSASANA (head to knee posture)

Sit on the floor with your legs extended in front of the body. Bend your left knee and place the sole of your left foot against your right thigh. (If your knee doesn't touch the floor, support it with a cushion or a blanket.) Inhaling, straighten your spine and extend both hands to hold your right foot. (If you can't reach your foot, place a belt around it and hold the belt.) Exhaling, and keeping the spine straight, gently lower your trunk onto your right leg, making sure that the knee is kept locked (see opposite). Hold for as long as is comfortable. Then, inhaling, raise your trunk back to sitting posture. Repeat on the opposite side.

Two triangles of light are formed with this posture. The first is with the minor chakra halfway along each clavicle bone and with the minor chakra on the palm of each hand.

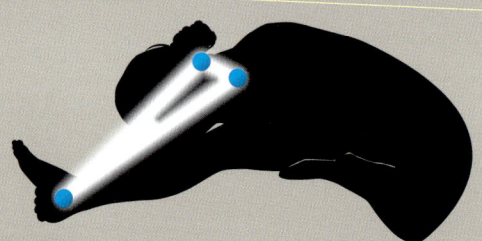

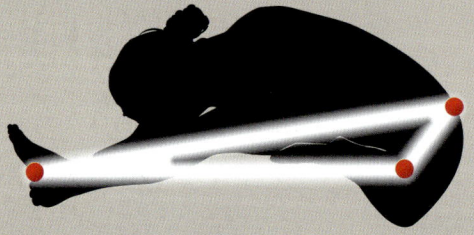

The second triangle is formed with the minor chakra on the sole of the extended foot, the minor chakra on the bent knee and the base chakra.

This posture stretches the hamstring muscles and loosens the hip joints. It removes excess fat in the abdominal region, tones the abdominal muscles and can relieve diabetes by working with the pancreas. Janu sirsasana also activates the kidneys, liver and adrenal glands, and encourages a good flow of blood to the spinal nerves and muscles. The posture is considered a powerful asana for spiritual awakening. The main chakra it works with is the sacral chakra.

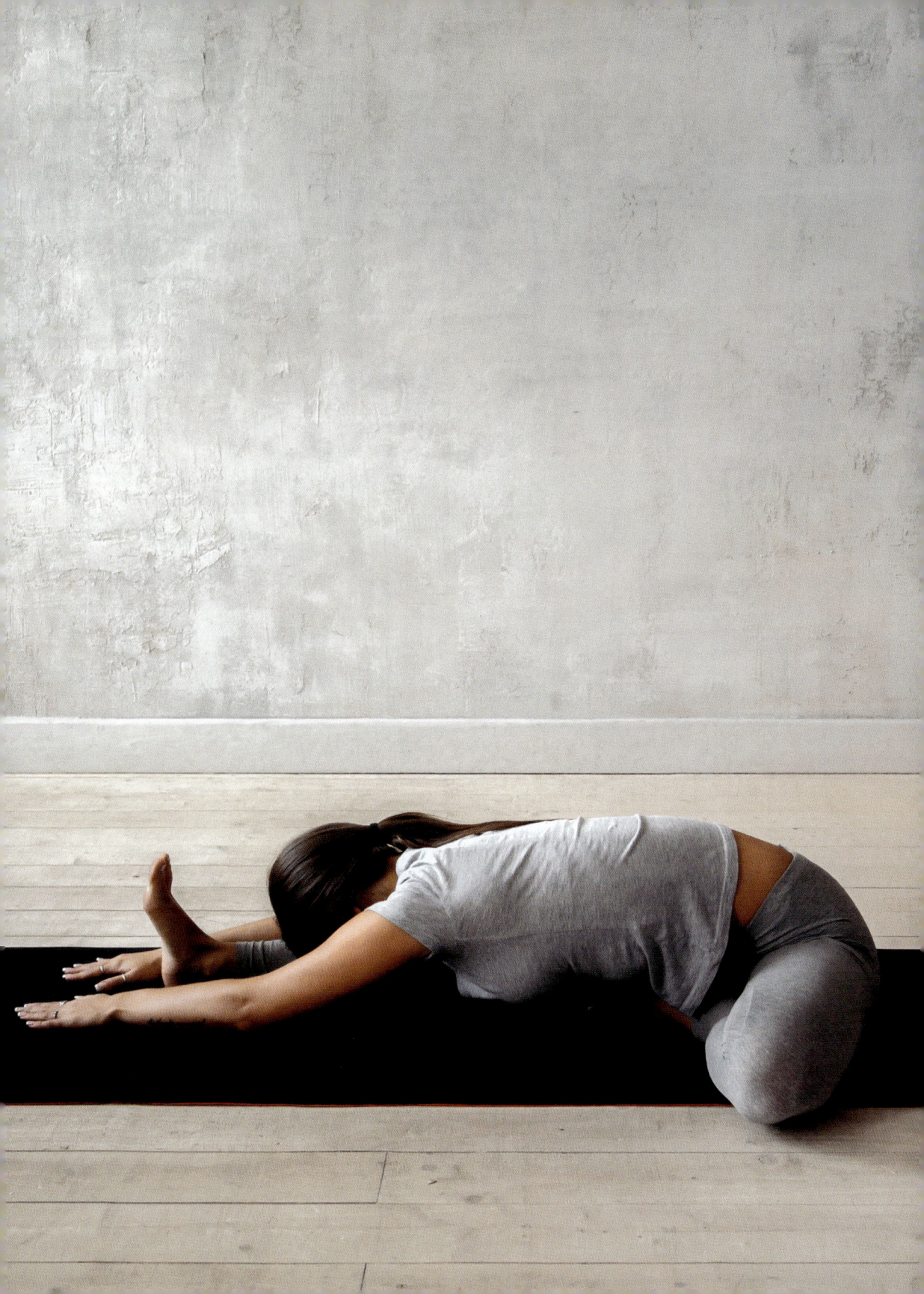

UPAVISTHA KONASANA (angle posture)

Sit on the floor, with your legs spread as wide as possible. Raise your arms over your head, keeping them straight, and clasp your hands. Turn your body towards your right leg. On an inhalation, lift your body, thus straightening the spine. While exhaling, gently lower your body onto your right leg, keeping the knee locked and making sure that the left buttock doesn't lose contact with the floor (see opposite). On the next inhalation, return to sitting posture. Turn your body towards your left leg and, while exhaling, lower your body down to your left leg. Inhale, and raise your trunk back to sitting posture. If you can't touch your foot with your hands, hold onto a belt placed around the foot.

This posture stretches the hamstring muscles and helps the blood to circulate in the pelvic region. It helps to prevent the development of a hernia, relieves sciatic pains, regularizes menstruation and stimulates the ovaries. The main chakra the posture activates is the sacral chakra.

Two main triangles of light are created in this posture. The first is with the sacral chakra and the minor chakra on the sole of each foot.

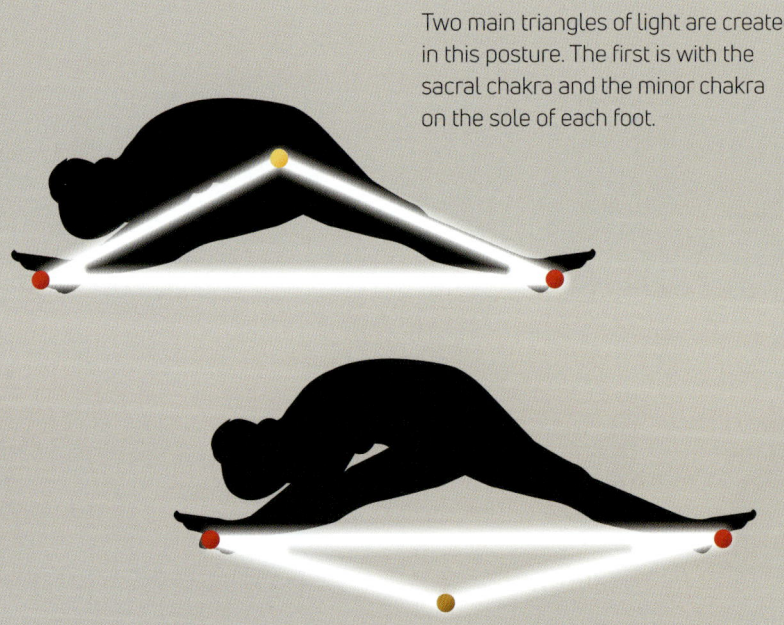

The second triangle is formed with the minor chakra on the sole of each foot and the earth chakra 15–20 cm (6–8 in) below the feet. As you hold the posture, visualize either or both of the triangles filling with white pranic energy.

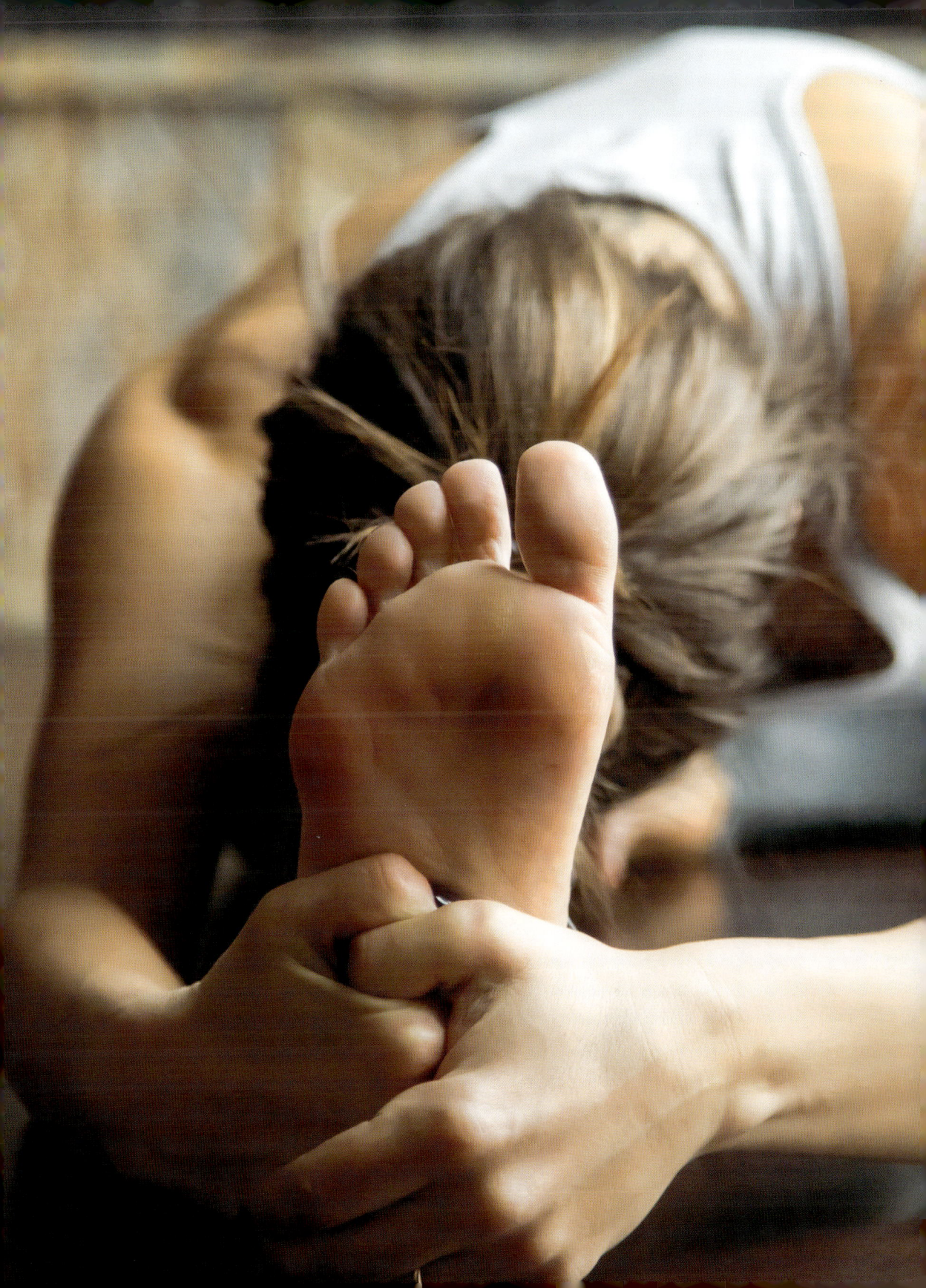

PURVOTTANASANA (upward plank posture)

Sit on the floor, with your legs stretched out in front. Place the palms of your hands on the floor, by the hips, with the fingers pointing towards your feet. Bend your knees, placing the soles of the feet on the floor. Exhale, pushing down with your hands and feet to lift your trunk off the floor. Keeping your arms straight, straighten your legs, raising the buttocks as high as possible. Take your head back (see opposite).

This intense body stretch strengthens the wrists and ankles, and works on the shoulder joints and hips. The chest is fully expanded, which is good way to open the heart chakra. Purvottanasana works with both the heart and throat chakras.

Four triangles of light are formed in this posture. The first is with the heart chakra and the minor chakra on the palm of each hand.

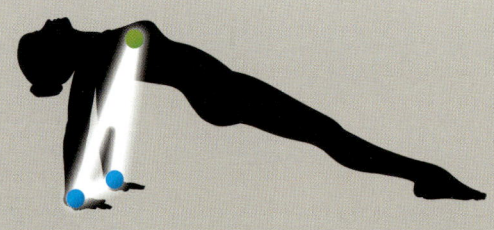

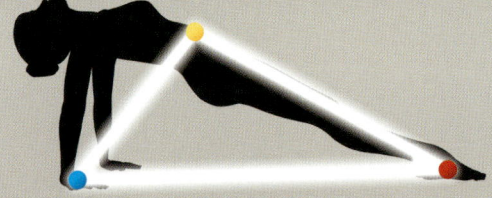

The second triangle is created with the solar plexus chakra, the minor chakra on the palm of the hand and the minor chakra on the sole of the foot.

The third triangle encompasses the throat chakra, the minor chakra on the sole of the foot and the minor chakra on the palm of the hand.

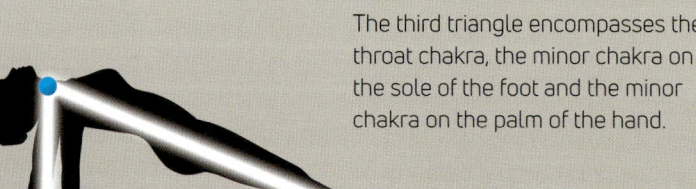

The fourth triangle is with the soul star chakra, the heart chakra and the minor chakra on the palm of the hand. All triangles of light, except the first, appear on both sides of the body.

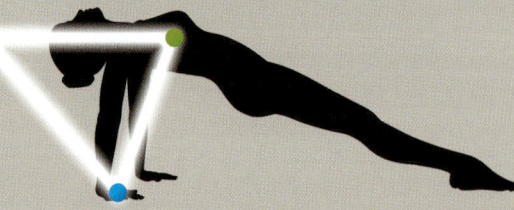

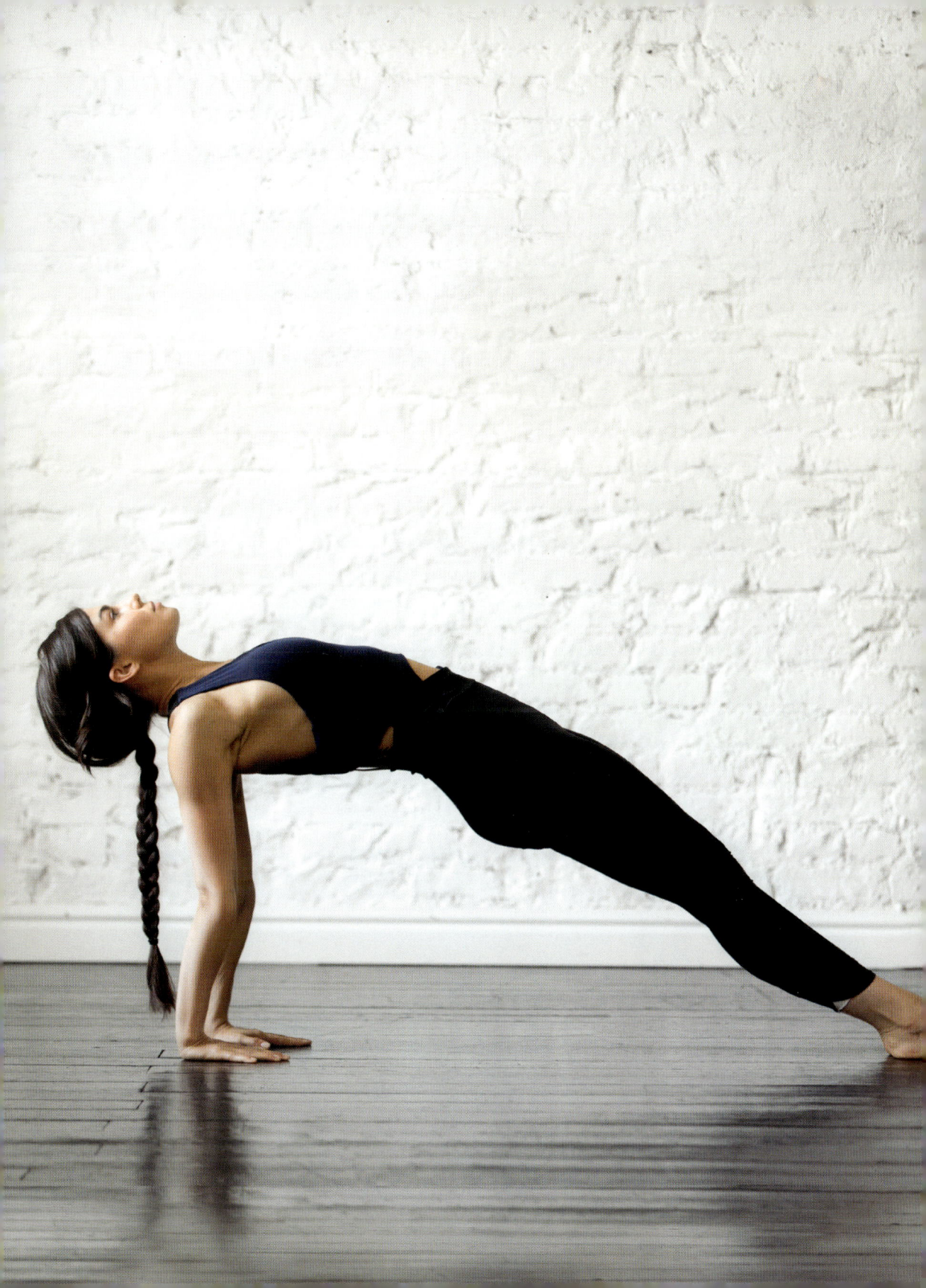

ARDHA MATSYENDRASANA
(half spinal twist)

Sit on the floor, with your legs stretched out in front of you. Bend your left knee, taking your right leg over the left leg and placing the sole of the right foot on the floor beside the left knee. Bend your left knee, placing the heel of your foot by the right buttock. Turn your trunk towards the right leg, taking your left arm over your right knee. Place the palm of your right hand on the floor, behind and close to your body, with the fingers facing away from the body. Keeping both buttocks on the floor, on the next exhalation rotate your trunk as far to the right as possible, looking over your right shoulder (see opposite). Try to imagine that you have a wall behind you, and your aim is to place your back and both shoulders against the wall. Hold this posture for as long as is comfortable. On an inhalation, return to the starting position and then repeat on the opposite side.

   This posture makes the spine and back muscles supple. It massages the abdominal organs and aids digestion. It tones the kidneys, adrenal glands and pancreas – so is beneficial for people suffering from diabetes. The main chakra the posture works with is the solar plexus chakra.

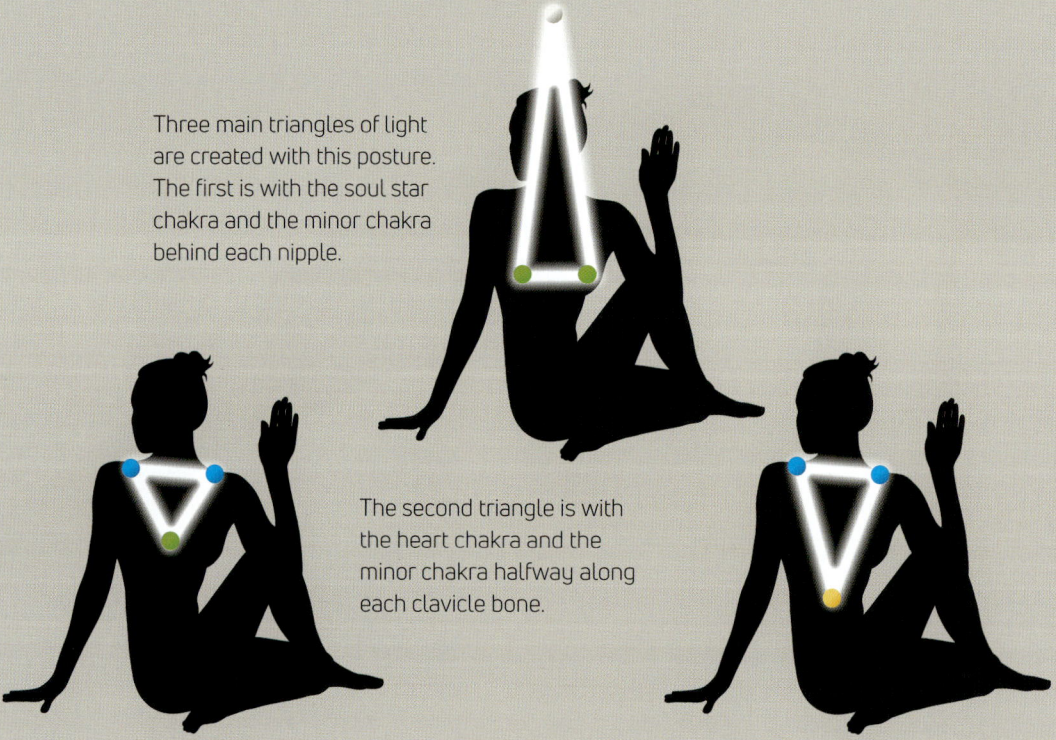

Three main triangles of light are created with this posture. The first is with the soul star chakra and the minor chakra behind each nipple.

The second triangle is with the heart chakra and the minor chakra halfway along each clavicle bone.

The third triangle is formed with the solar plexus chakra and the minor chakra halfway along each clavicle bone.

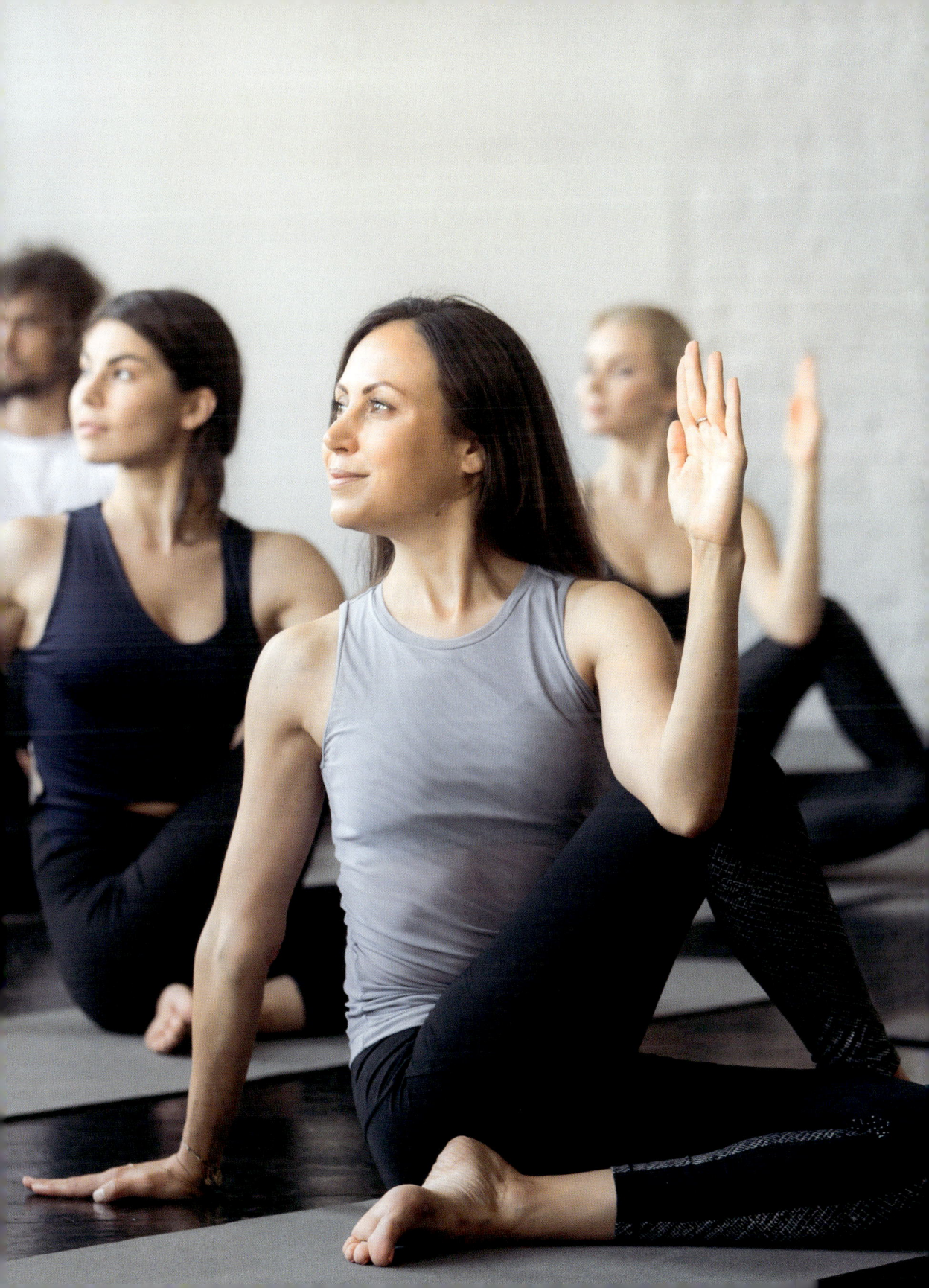

NAVASANA (boat posture)

Sit on the floor, with your legs stretched out in front of you, keeping your spine straight. Place the palms of your hands on the floor by your hips, with your fingers pointing towards your feet. Exhale, and recline your trunk slightly back, simultaneously raising your legs from the floor. Bring your feet in line with your head, keeping the legs straight and your knees locked. Stretch your arms forwards, keeping them parallel to the floor and close to your body (see opposite). Hold the posture for as long as possible. If you find navasana difficult, you can place your head against a wall for support.

This asana reduces fat around the waistline, tones the kidneys, gall bladder, liver and spleen, and works on the thighs and abdominal muscles. It also improves balance, reduces nervous tension and aids poor digestion. The main chakra it works with is the base chakra.

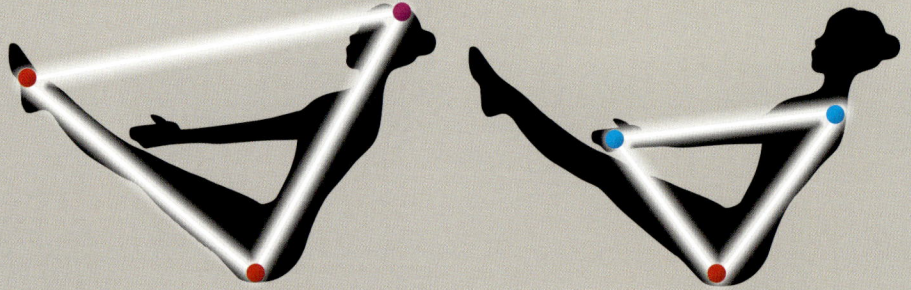

Three main triangles of light are activated in this posture. The first is formed with the crown chakra, the minor chakra on the sole of the foot and the base chakra. The second triangle is created with the minor chakra halfway along the clavicle bone, the minor chakra on the palm of the hand and the base chakra.

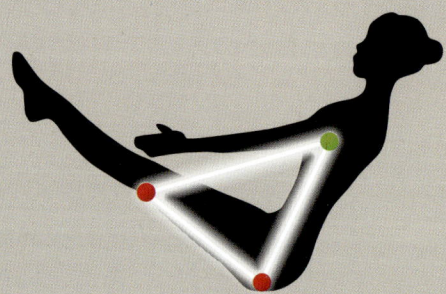

The third triangle arises from the heart chakra, the minor chakra behind the knee and the base chakra. All three triangles are formed on both sides of the body.

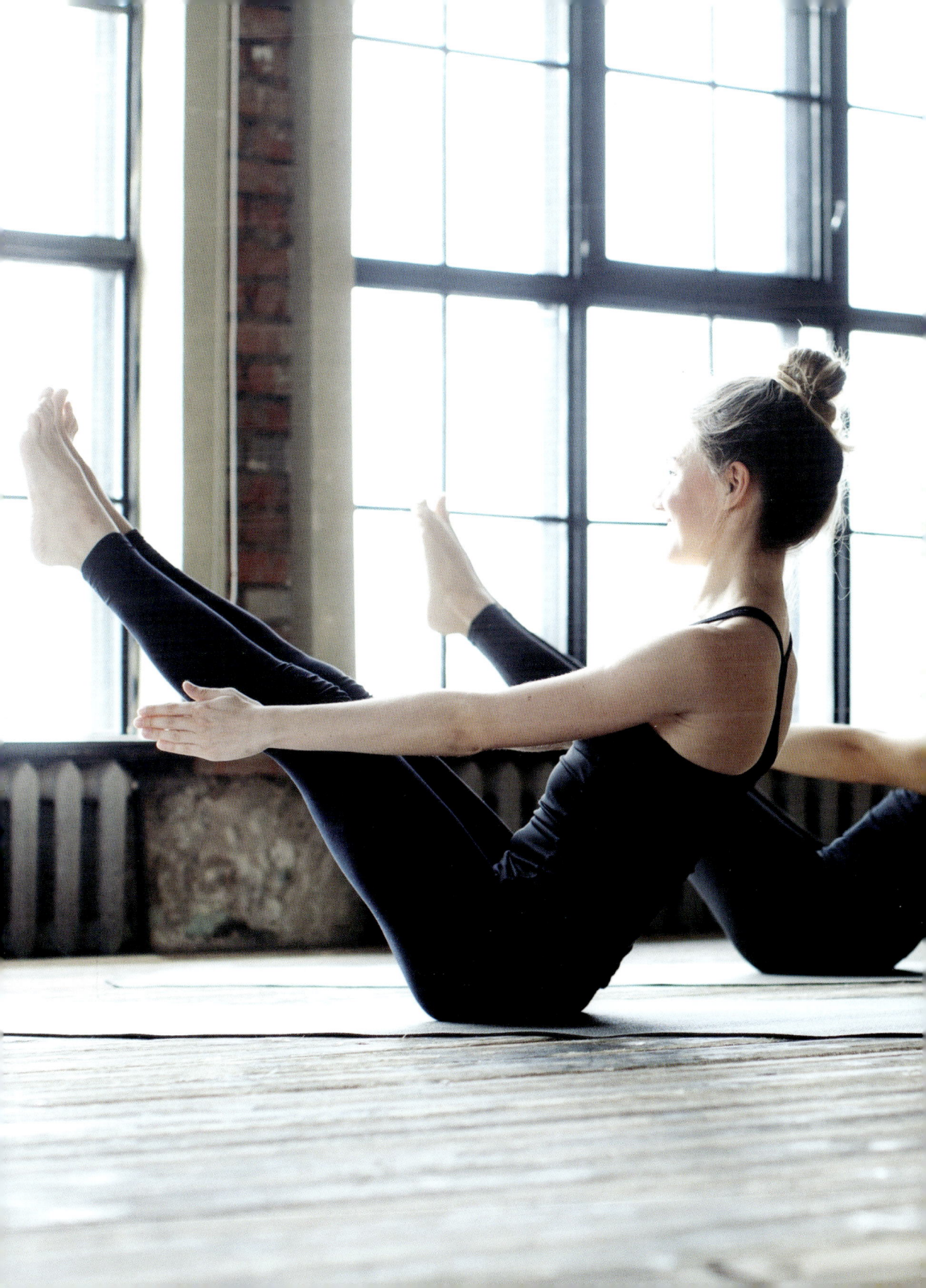

ANAHATA ASANA (heart posture)

Start on all fours. Then, on the next inhalation, extend your arms forwards until
your chin and chest touch the floor. As you exhale, extend the end of your coccyx
upwards to allow your shoulders to come closer to the floor (see opposite).
If you can't get your chest and chin onto the floor, you can begin by placing
your forehead on the floor.

This asana benefits the heart chakra by opening the chest cavity. It also
stretches the chest, shoulder and back muscles.

There are three main triangles of light
present in this posture. The first is
created with the minor chakra in the
palm of the hand, the base chakra and
the minor chakra on the sole of the foot.

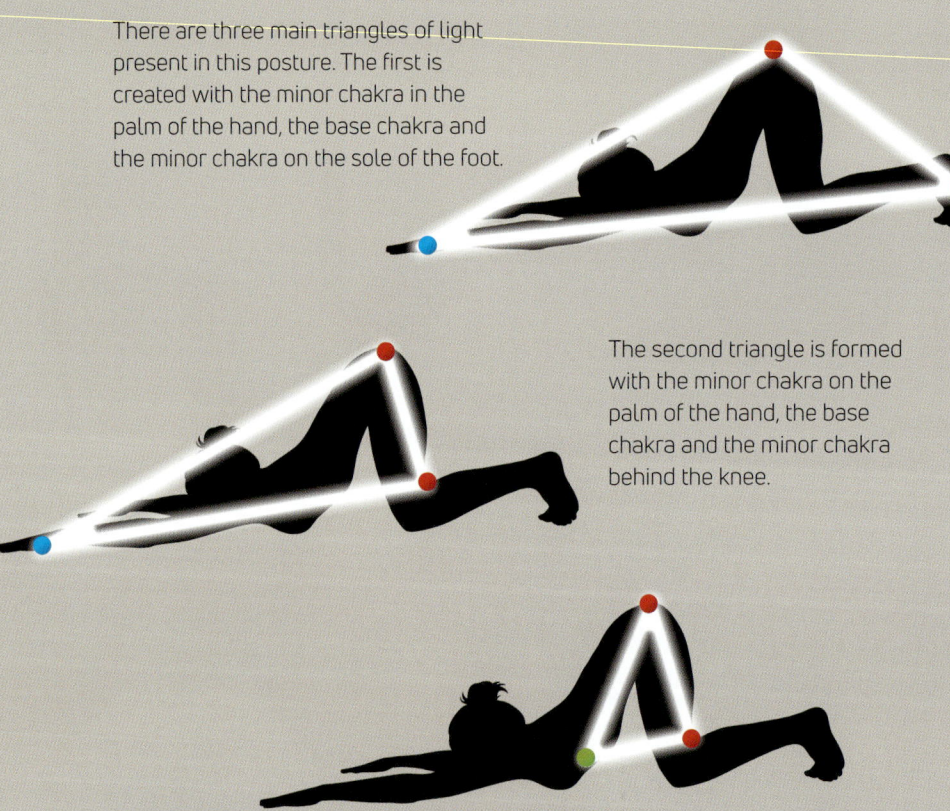

The second triangle is formed
with the minor chakra on the
palm of the hand, the base
chakra and the minor chakra
behind the knee.

The third triangle arises from the heart chakra, the base chakra
and the minor chakra behind the knee. These three triangles
are formed on both sides of the body.

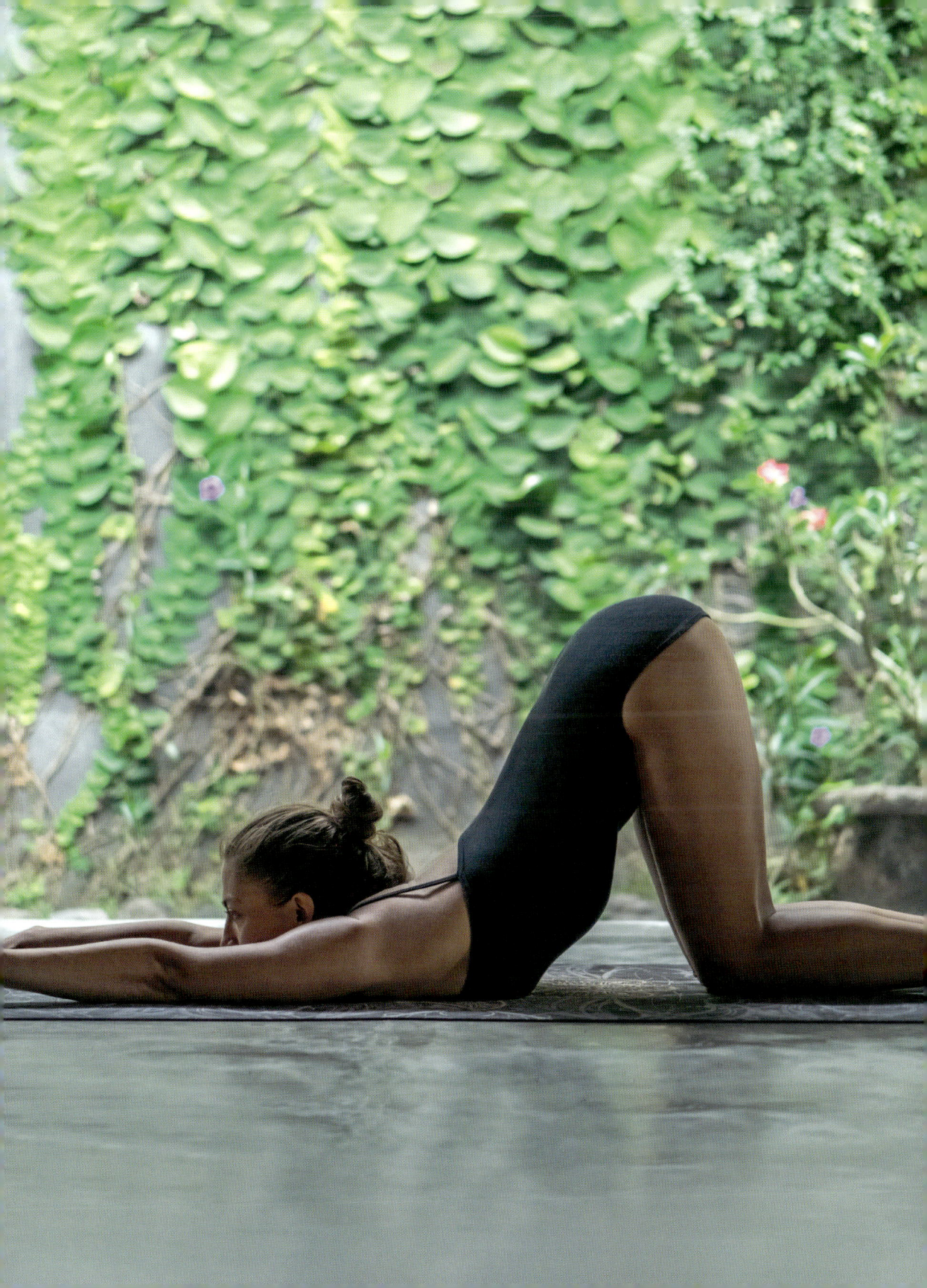

HANUMANASANA (the splits)

This is an advanced posture. Before attempting it, other postures should be practised to make the body supple.

Kneel on the floor. Bend your right knee, placing the sole of your foot on the floor. Place the palms of both hands on the floor on either side of your body. Gently slide your right leg forwards and left leg backwards, taking the weight of your body on your arms and hands. Keep extending your legs until they're straight and lying on the ground (see opposite). If at first your trunk doesn't touch the floor, you can place blankets or cushions underneath. Hanumanasana can take some time to master, but with regular practice it can be achieved.

The posture improves blood circulation in the legs, thighs and hips, and tones the leg muscles. It strengthens and relaxes the thigh abductor muscles and helps those suffering from sciatica. The main chakra activated is the base chakra.

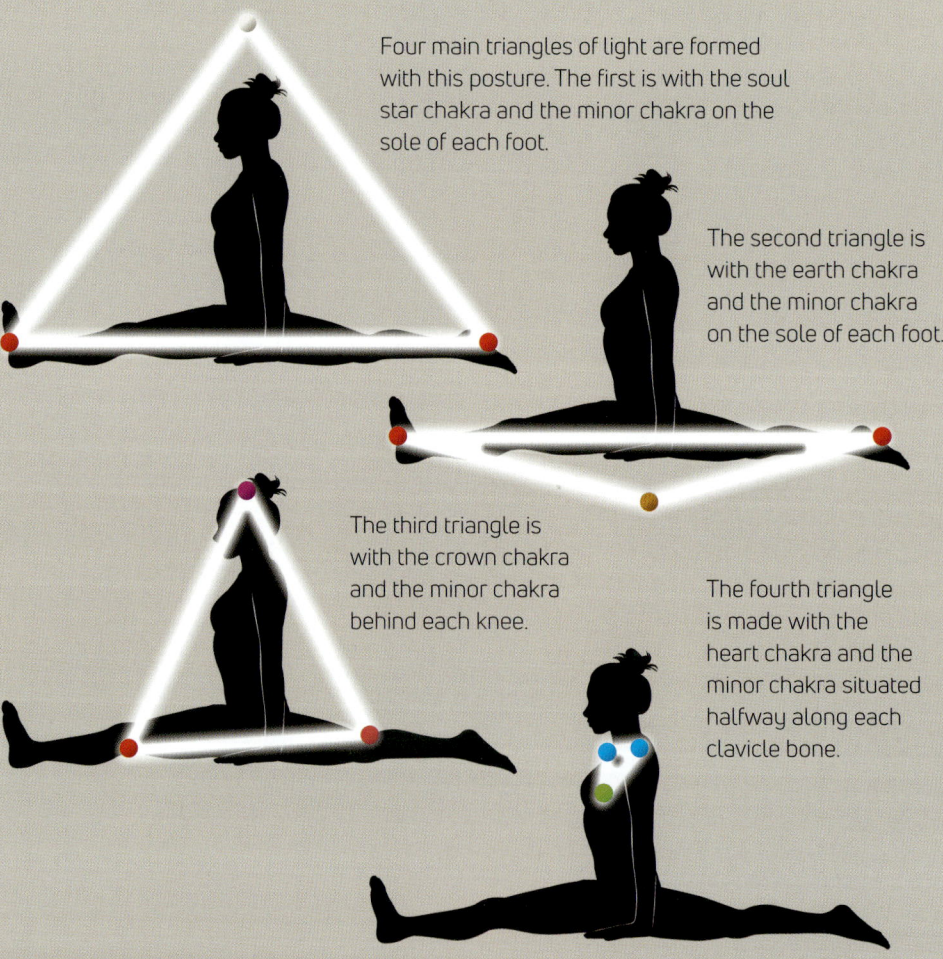

Four main triangles of light are formed with this posture. The first is with the soul star chakra and the minor chakra on the sole of each foot.

The second triangle is with the earth chakra and the minor chakra on the sole of each foot.

The third triangle is with the crown chakra and the minor chakra behind each knee.

The fourth triangle is made with the heart chakra and the minor chakra situated halfway along each clavicle bone.

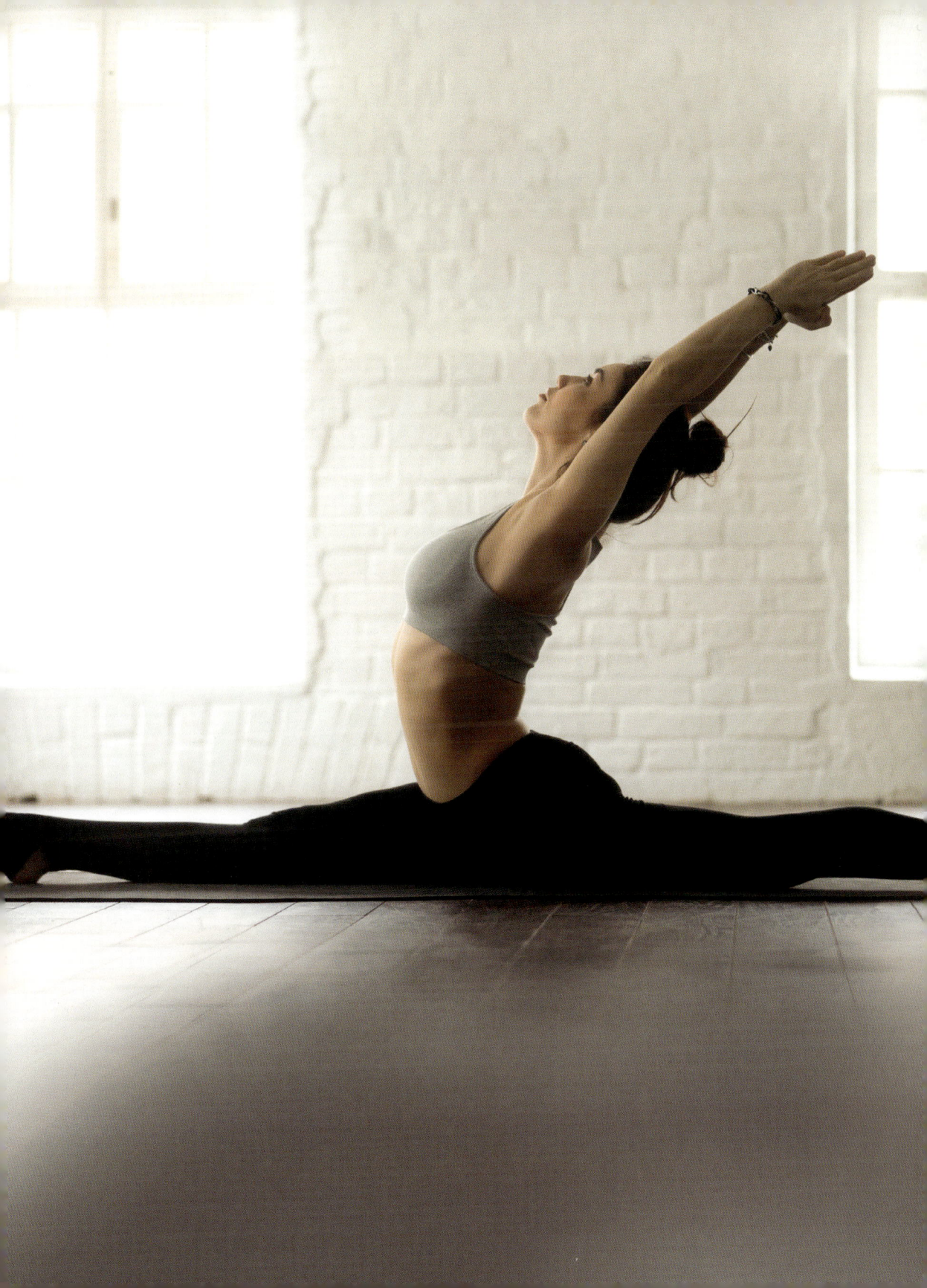

UTTHITA HASTA PADANGUSTHASANA
(extended hand to toe posture)

If you need support when you first work with this posture, it can be practised against a wall or lying on the floor. If you can't reach your foot with your hand, put a belt around your foot.

Stand either in the middle of the floor, against a wall or lying on the floor. Bend your left knee and hold your foot with your left hand or place a belt around your foot, holding the end of the belt at a position that's comfortable for you. Now straighten the leg out in front of you.

Holding the belt or foot with your left hand, gently take your leg out to the side of your body and raise your right arm so that it's in line with your left arm (see opposite). Hold for as long as is comfortable and then change over legs.

This asana stretches the hamstring muscles, strengthens the leg joints and muscles, and helps to maintain balance.

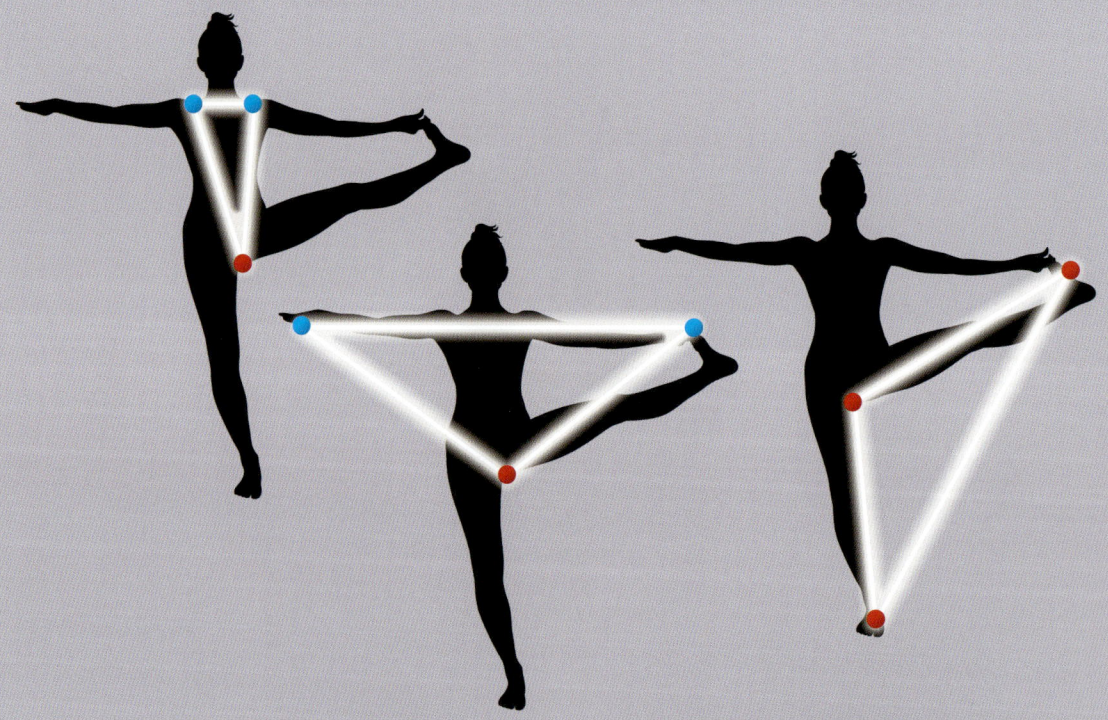

Three main triangles of light are formed in this posture. The first (left) is with the base chakra and the minor chakra halfway along each clavicle bone. The second triangle (centre) arises from the base chakra and the minor chakra on the palm of each hand. The third triangle (right) is created with the base chakra and the minor chakra on the sole of each foot. Work either with all three triangles or with one triangle at a time.

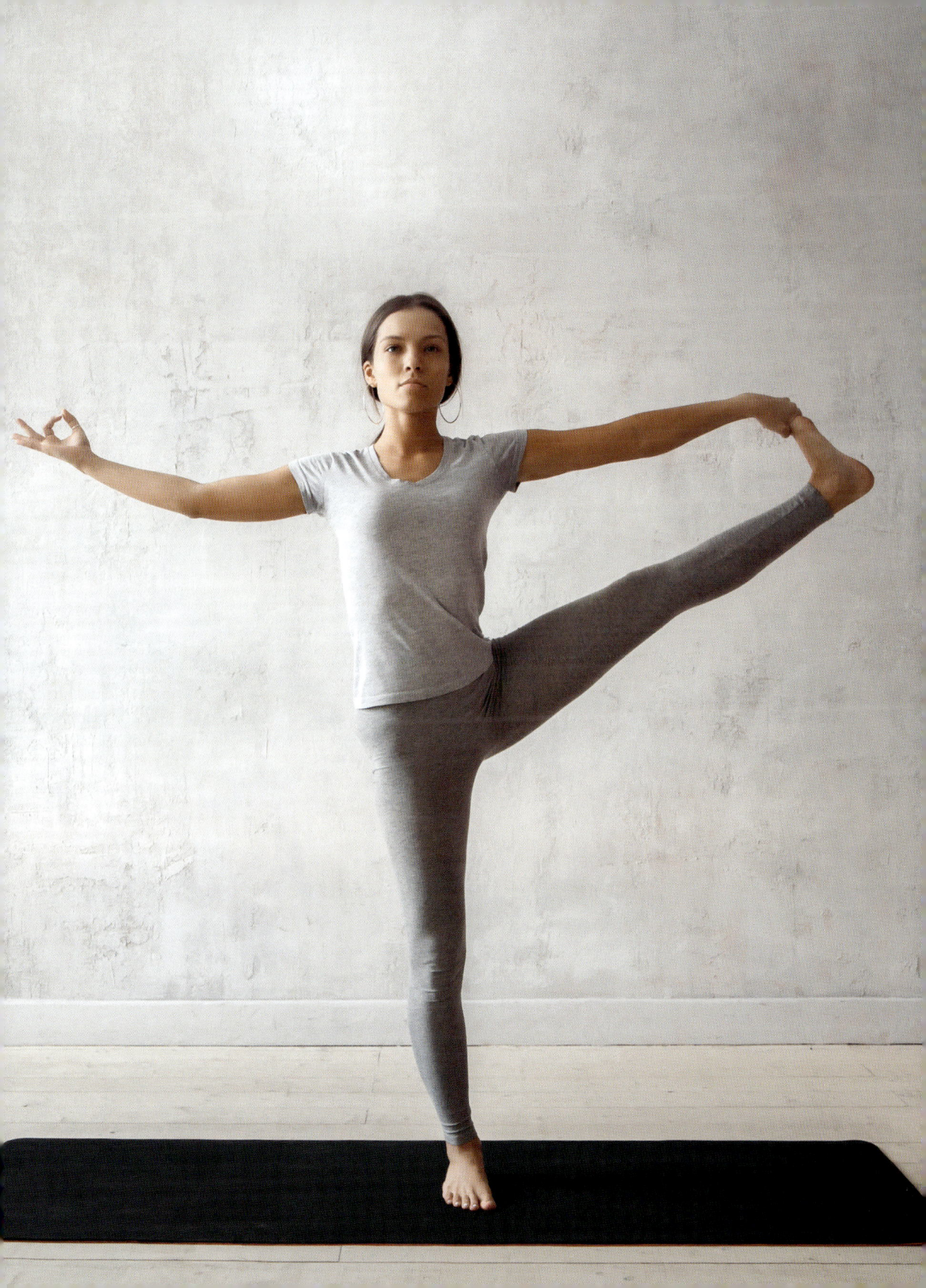

ADHO MUKHA SVANASANA (dog posture)

Lie face down on the floor, with your feet about 30 cm (1 ft) apart. Bend your elbows and place your hands on the floor, level with your breasts. Tuck your toes under and come into a kneeling position. Push down with your hands, straighten your legs and lower your heels onto the floor. If the heels don't touch the floor, place either a blanket or book under them. Curve your back inwards, and slowly bring your head down towards the floor (see opposite). Make sure that your knees and elbows are kept locked.

In the dog posture, the whole of the back is stretched, and the muscles of the shoulders are relaxed. The legs, ankles, arms and wrists are strengthened, and the nervous system is stimulated, supplying fresh energy to the body. The posture works with the base chakra.

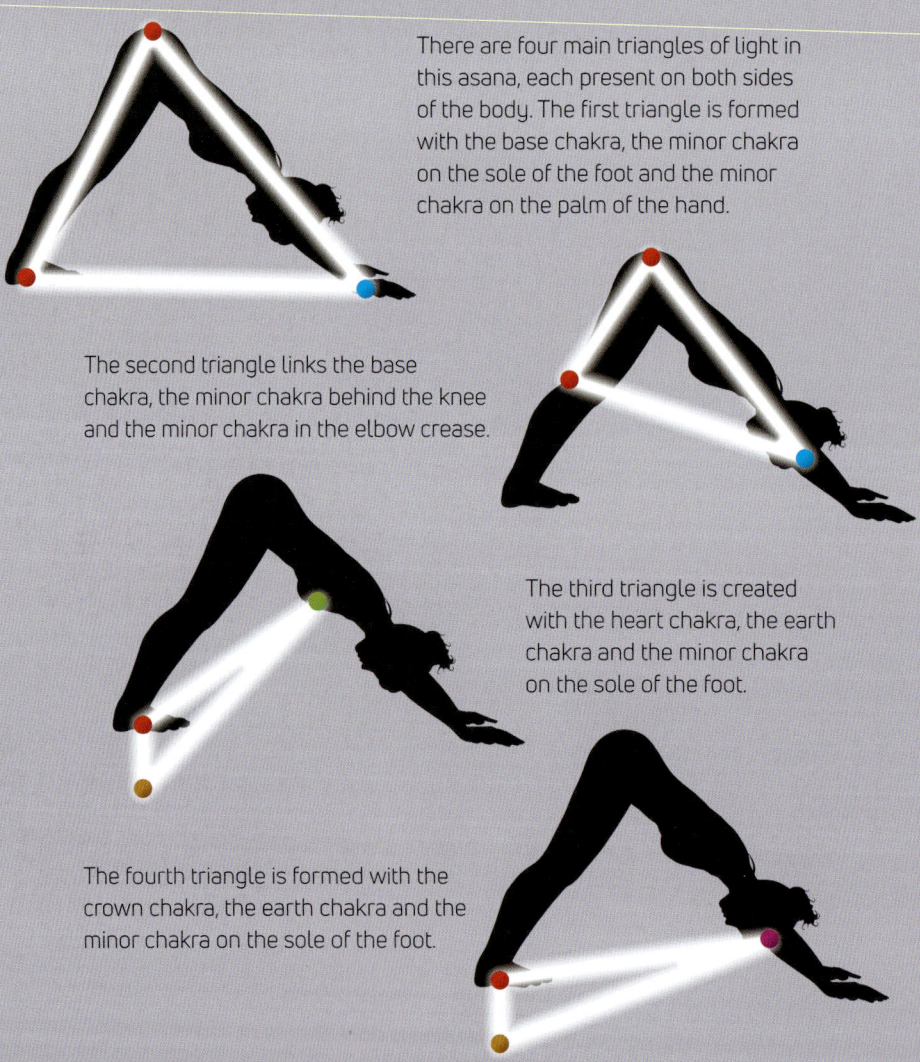

There are four main triangles of light in this asana, each present on both sides of the body. The first triangle is formed with the base chakra, the minor chakra on the sole of the foot and the minor chakra on the palm of the hand.

The second triangle links the base chakra, the minor chakra behind the knee and the minor chakra in the elbow crease.

The third triangle is created with the heart chakra, the earth chakra and the minor chakra on the sole of the foot.

The fourth triangle is formed with the crown chakra, the earth chakra and the minor chakra on the sole of the foot.

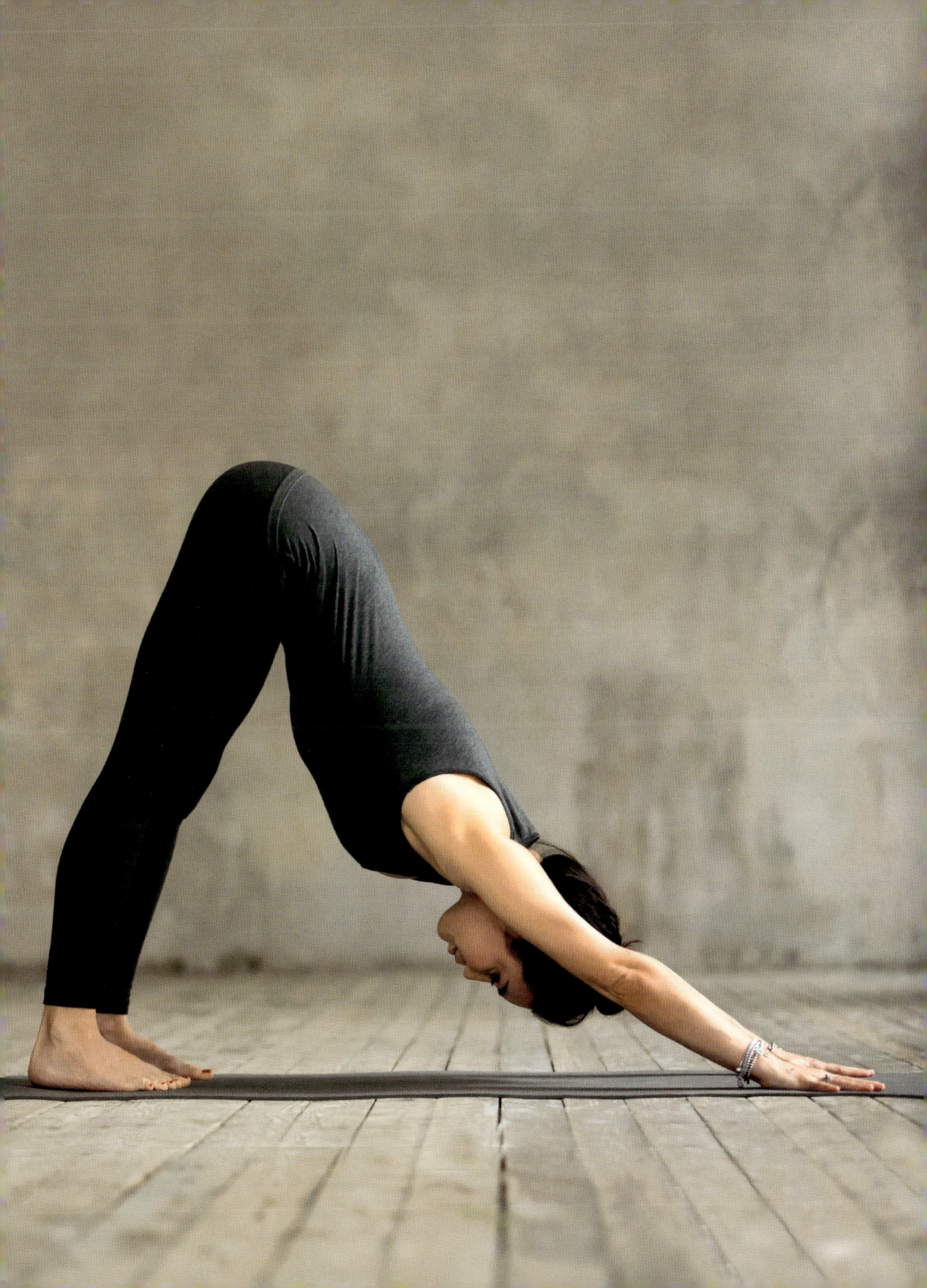

TRIKONASANA (triangle posture)

Standing upright, walk your feet about 1 m (3 ft) apart. Turn your right foot
90 degrees and turn your left foot slightly towards your right foot. Adjust your
feet so that the heel of the right foot is in line with the arch of the left foot. Extend
both arms horizontally, then bend sideways, taking your right arm down and
placing your hand as far down your left leg as possible. Eventually, with practice,
the right hand can be placed on the floor by the outside of the right foot (see
opposite). Extend your left arm upwards, palm facing forwards. Rotate your trunk
from the hips to open your chest. Turn your head to look up at the upstretched
arm. To ensure that the position of the body is correct, this posture can be done
against a wall. If you use a wall, when you rotate your trunk, your back and both
shoulders should touch the wall.

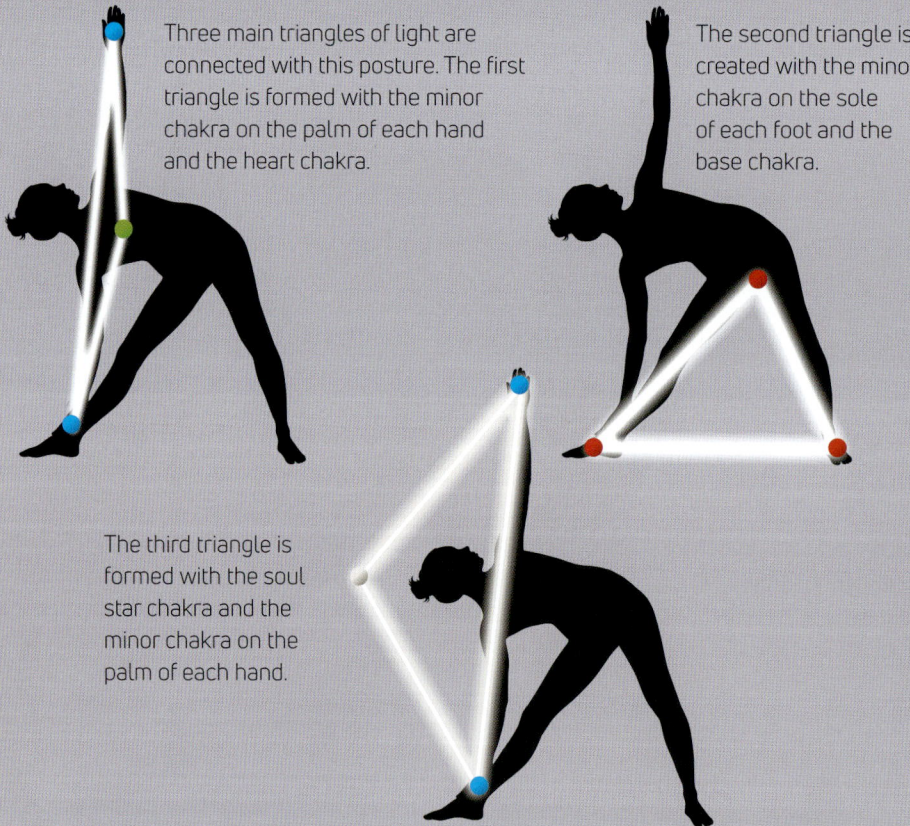

Three main triangles of light are
connected with this posture. The first
triangle is formed with the minor
chakra on the palm of each hand
and the heart chakra.

The second triangle is
created with the minor
chakra on the sole
of each foot and the
base chakra.

The third triangle is
formed with the soul
star chakra and the
minor chakra on the
palm of each hand.

This asana works on the hamstring muscles and thighs. It fully expands the chest,
invigorates the abdominal organs and strengthens the hip muscles. The main
chakra activated by trikonasana is the heart chakra.

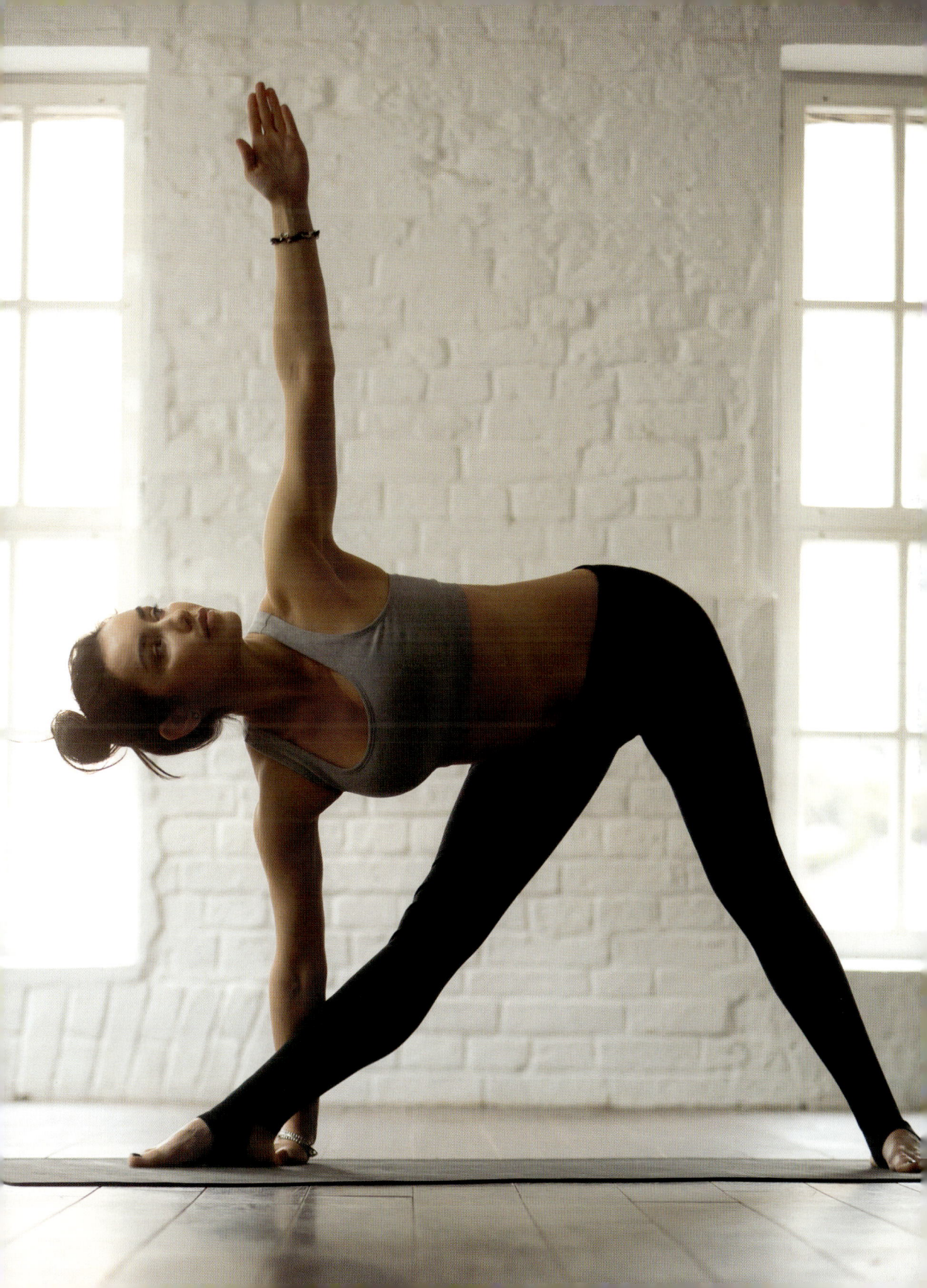

PARIVRTTA TRIKONASANA
(revolving triangle posture)

Stand upright, with your feet together, spine straight and shoulders back. Inhale, and either jump or walk the feet about 1 m (3 ft) apart. Turn both feet 90 degrees to the left so your body is facing to the left, with your feet and hips in line. Inhale, and rotate your trunk to the left. Take your right hand over your left leg and onto the floor. Stretch your left arm up until it's in line with the right arm, fully expanding your chest (see opposite). Keep both knees locked and look up at your right hand. Hold for as long as is comfortable, then, on an inhalation, come back to standing posture. If you can't touch the floor, place your hand on a yoga brick or a pile of books by the outside of the left foot. Repeat the posture on the opposite side.

If you find it hard to balance in this posture, it can be done against a wall. Place the left side of your body against the wall, then take your right foot forwards and your left hand over your right foot. The aim is to place your back and shoulders against the wall, fully opening your chest. Repeat the asana on the other side. The main chakra activated in revolving triangle posture is the heart chakra.

This posture works on the hamstring muscles and thighs. It fully expands the chest and aids concentration and balance. It invigorates the abdominal organs and strengthens the hip muscles.

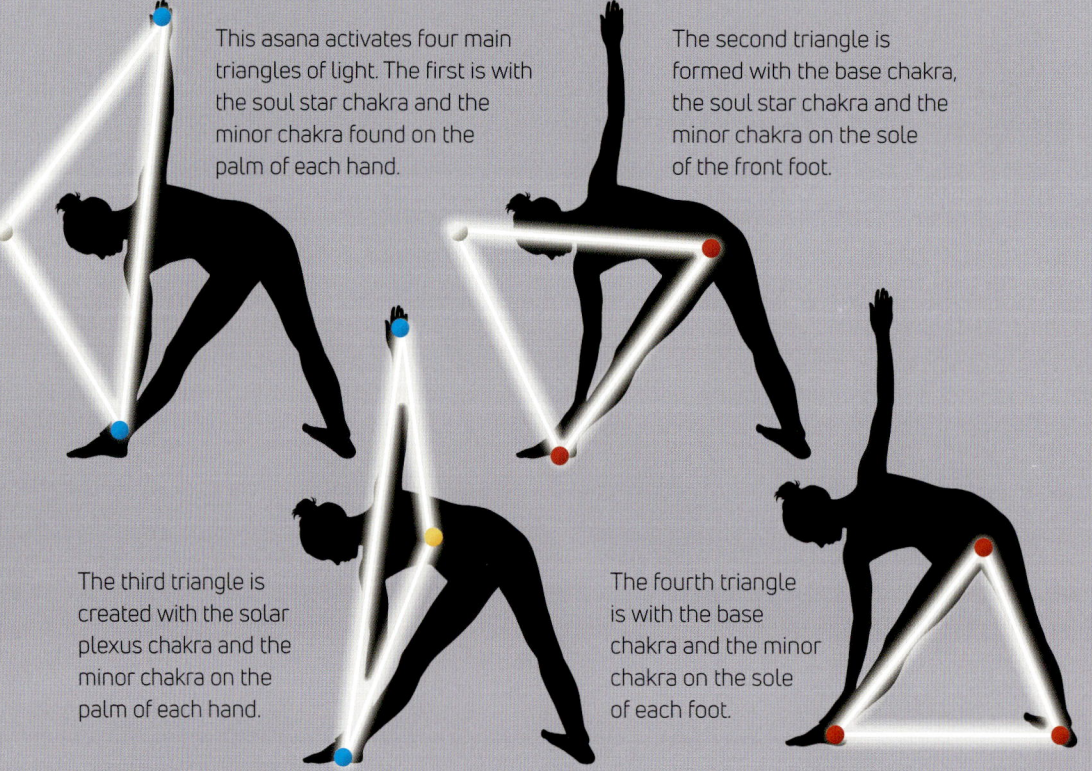

This asana activates four main triangles of light. The first is with the soul star chakra and the minor chakra found on the palm of each hand.

The second triangle is formed with the base chakra, the soul star chakra and the minor chakra on the sole of the front foot.

The third triangle is created with the solar plexus chakra and the minor chakra on the palm of each hand.

The fourth triangle is with the base chakra and the minor chakra on the sole of each foot.

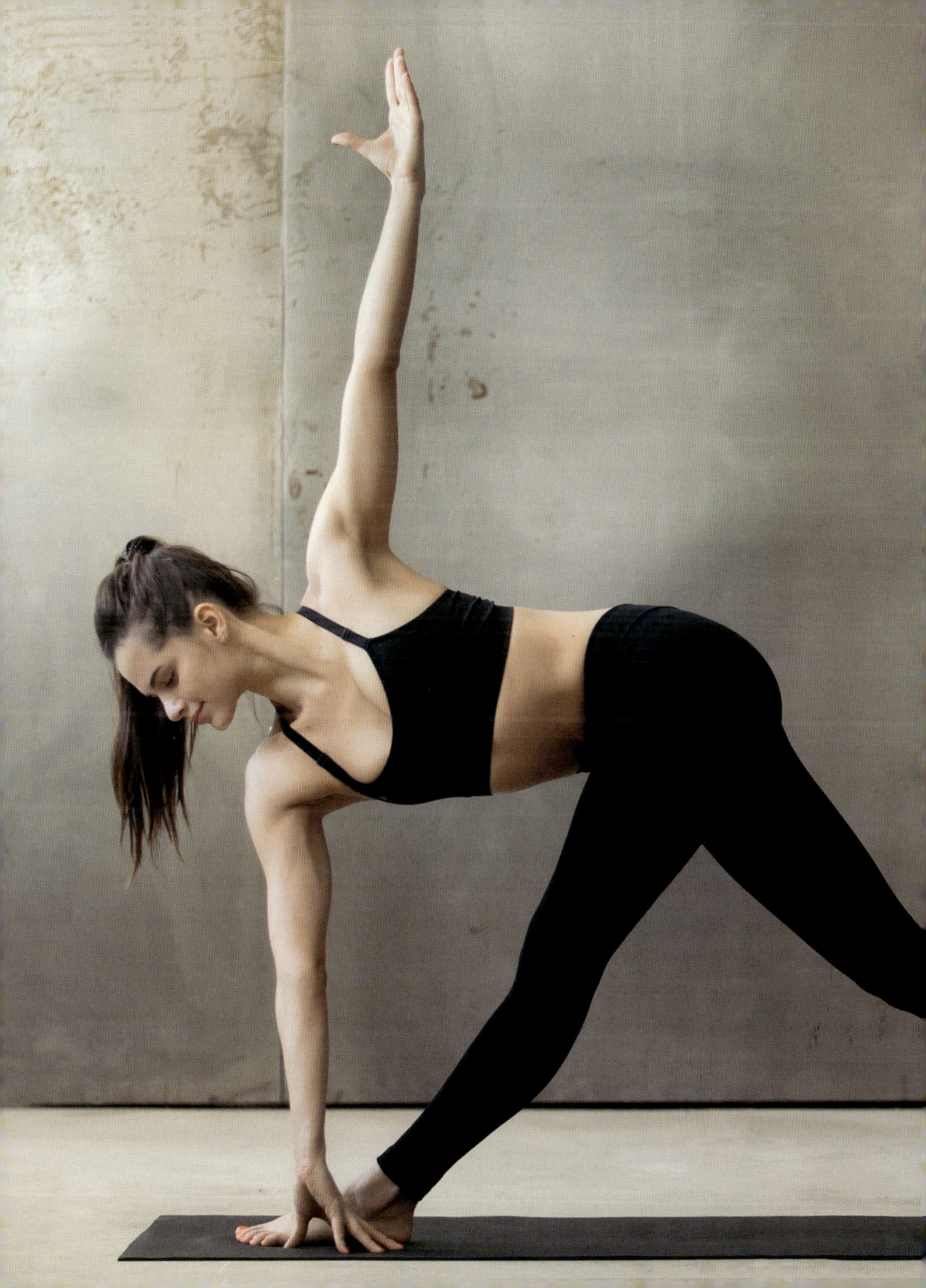

PRASARITA PADOTTANASANA
(expanded foot posture)

Stand upright, with your feet together, spine straight, shoulders back and chest expanded. Inhale, and jump or walk the feet about 1 m (3 ft) apart. Make sure that your feet are parallel and your toes in line. Exhaling, and keeping the spine straight, extend your trunk forwards from your hips, placing the palms of your hands on the ground, fingers facing forwards. If your hands can't reach the floor, place them on books or blankets. This is the intermediate posture.

Next, slowly walk your hands backwards until they're in line with your feet, at the same time extending your trunk until the top of your head rests on the floor, between the hands. Alternatively, the left hand can hold the left ankle and the right hand the right ankle (see opposite). Hold the posture for as long as is comfortable. Inhaling, come back to the intermediate position. Exhale and, on the next inhalation, return to the standing posture and bring your feet together.

Prasarita padottanasana works on the inner thigh and hamstring muscles, removes shoulder stiffness and fully opens the chest. A fresh supply of blood flows to the head, neck and trunk. This asana can be practised in place of the full head balance (see page 148). The main chakra activated is the crown chakra.

In this posture, one triangle is formed with the base chakra and the minor chakra on the sole of each foot, and another triangle with the soul star chakra and the minor chakra on the sole of each foot.

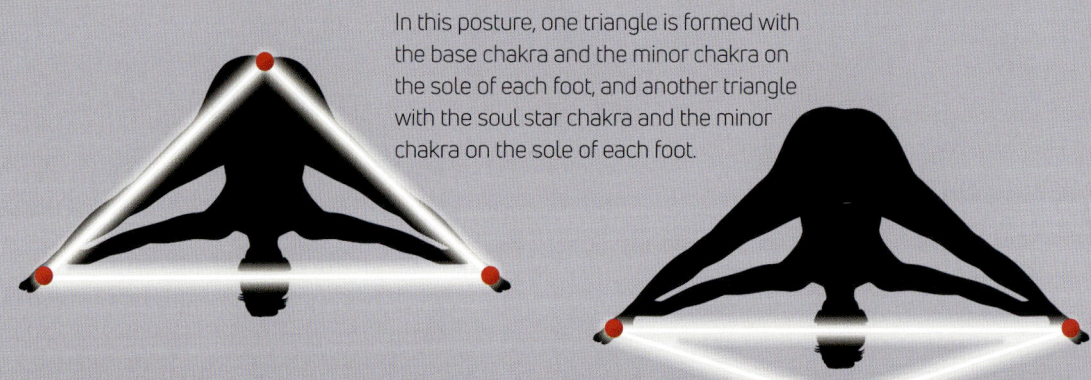

Three triangles are also formed in the head. The first is created with the crown chakra, the brow chakra and the alta major chakra. The second triangle is with the pineal gland, the pituitary gland and the carotid glands. The third head triangle is formed with the pituitary gland and the minor chakra behind each eye.

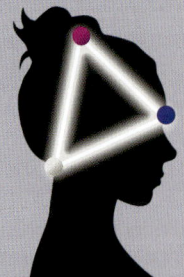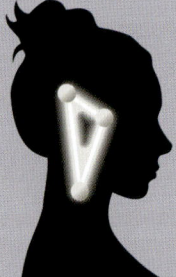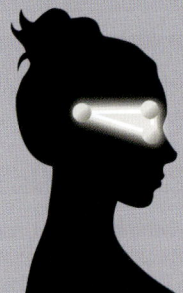

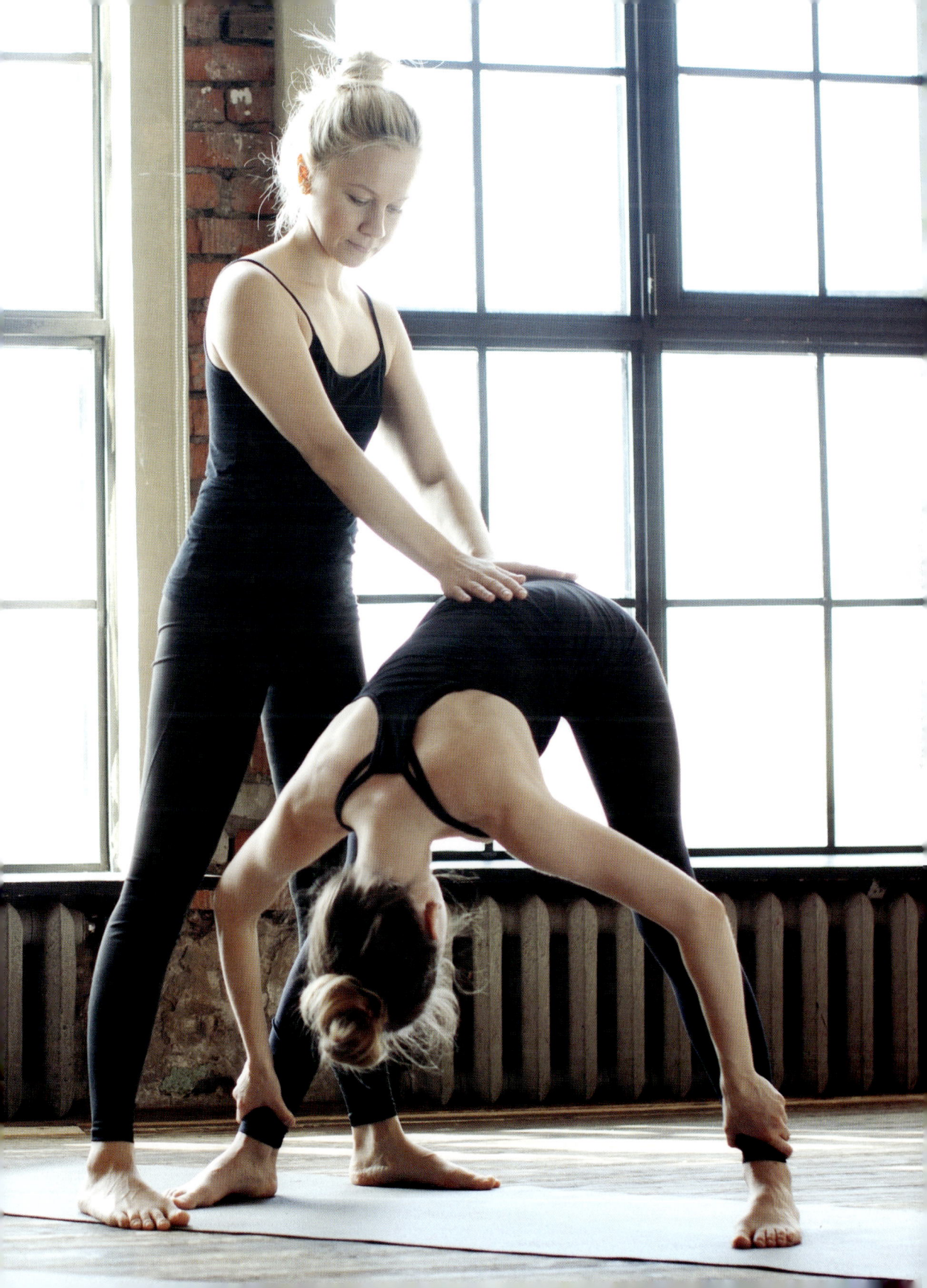

VIRABHADRASANA 1 (warrior posture 1)

Stand upright, with your feet together, spine straight and shoulders back. Inhale, and either jump or walk the feet about 1 m (3 ft) apart. Turn both feet to the left, making sure your pelvic girdle is straight. Bend your left knee until it's in line with the ankle, forming a right angle. Keeping your back leg straight, aim to place the heel of your right foot on the floor. Stretch both arms up over your head, keeping the arms straight, then join the palms of your hands (see opposite). Take your head back. Hold for as long as is comfortable before repeating on the other side.

Warrior posture 1 removes stiffness in the shoulders and back. It fully expands the chest, strengthens the ankles and knees, and reduces fat around the abdomen. The main chakra the asana works with is the heart chakra.

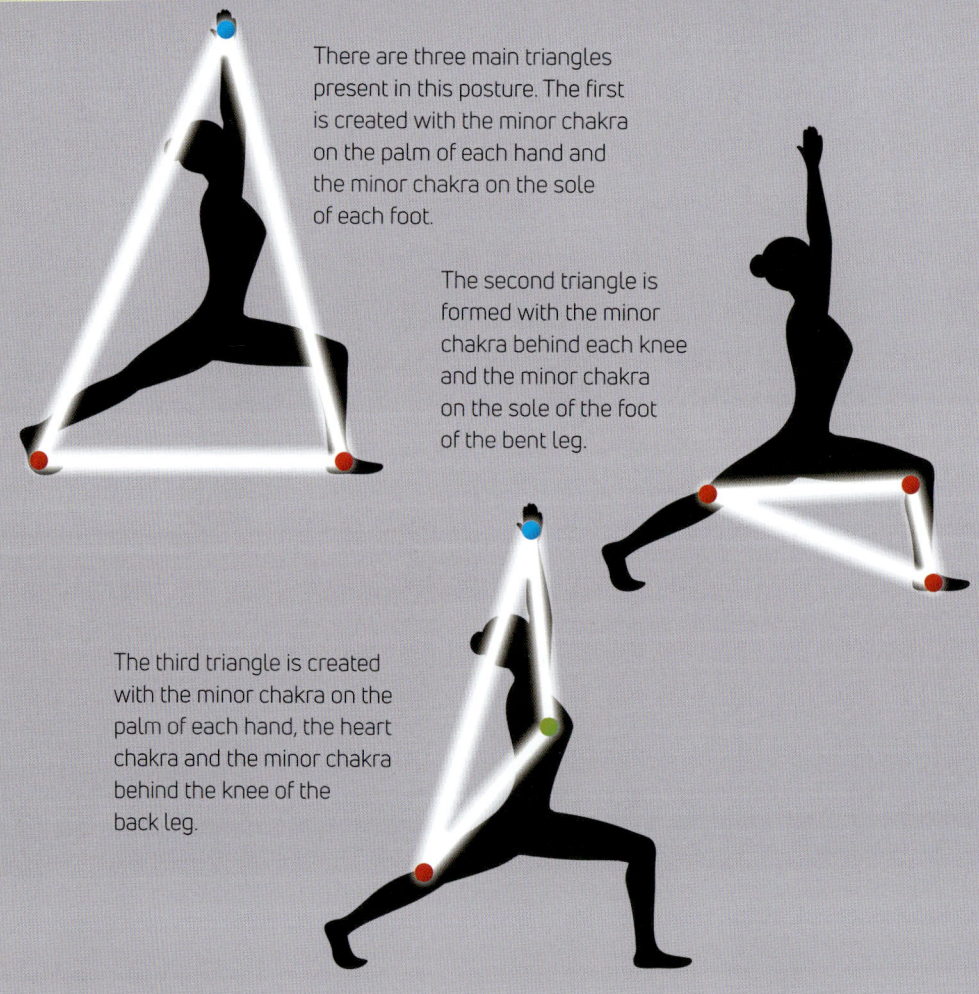

There are three main triangles present in this posture. The first is created with the minor chakra on the palm of each hand and the minor chakra on the sole of each foot.

The second triangle is formed with the minor chakra behind each knee and the minor chakra on the sole of the foot of the bent leg.

The third triangle is created with the minor chakra on the palm of each hand, the heart chakra and the minor chakra behind the knee of the back leg.

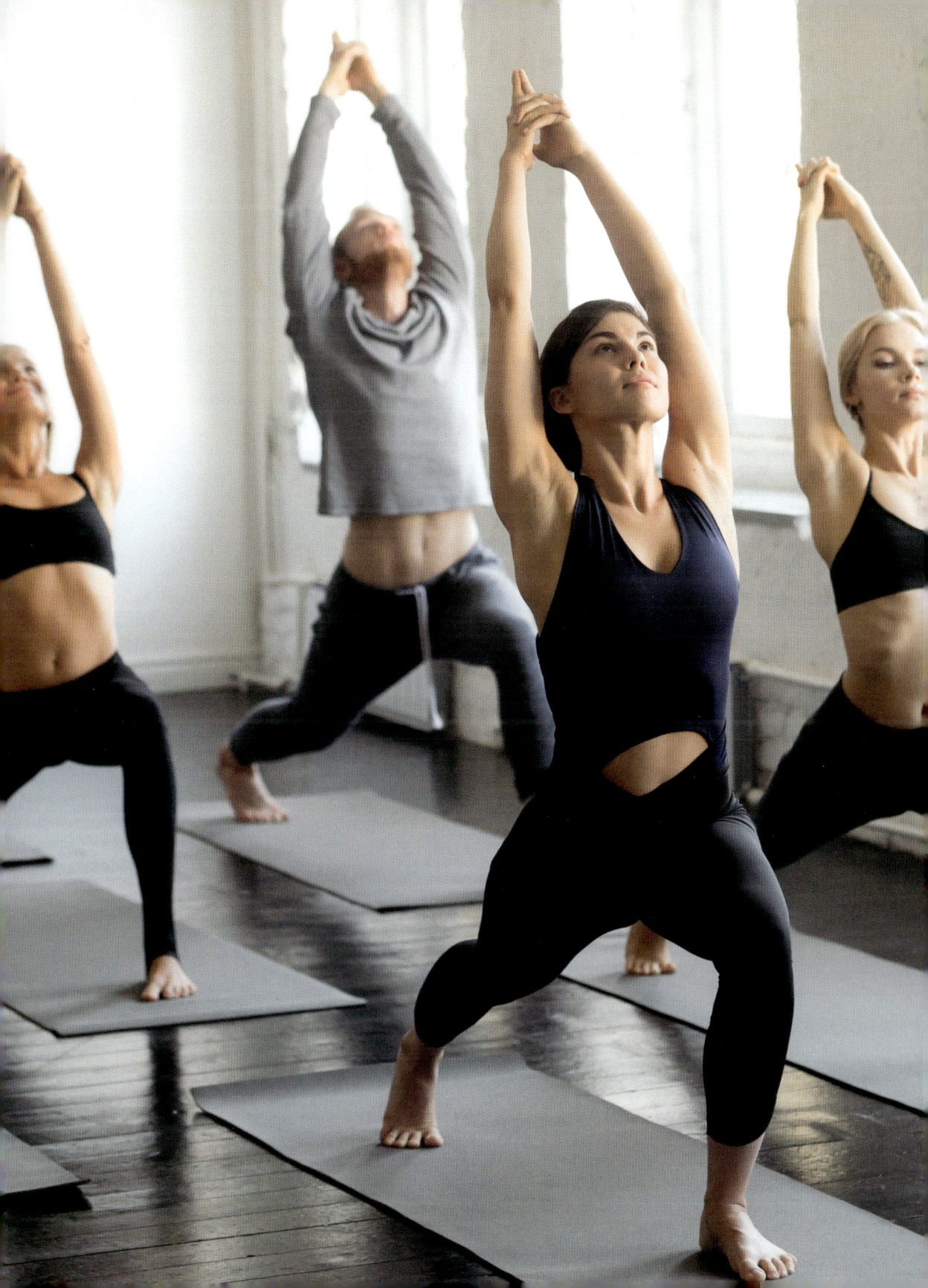

VIRABHADRASANA 2 (warrior posture 2)

Stand upright, with your feet together, spine straight and shoulders back. Inhale, and either jump or walk the feet approximately 1 m (3 ft) apart. Turn your left foot outwards 90 degrees, and your right foot slightly in, towards your left foot. Exhale, and bend your left knee, keeping it in line with your ankle and left hip. Extend your arms horizontally, feeling your chest opening. Turn your head towards your left hand (see opposite). Hold for as long as is comfortable, then, on the next inhalation, return to the standing position. Repeat on the opposite side.

Warrior posture 2 opens and expands the chest, allowing for deeper breathing. It strengthens the leg muscles, relieves cramp in the calf and thigh muscles, and helps to strengthen the whole body. The main chakra worked with the asana is the heart chakra.

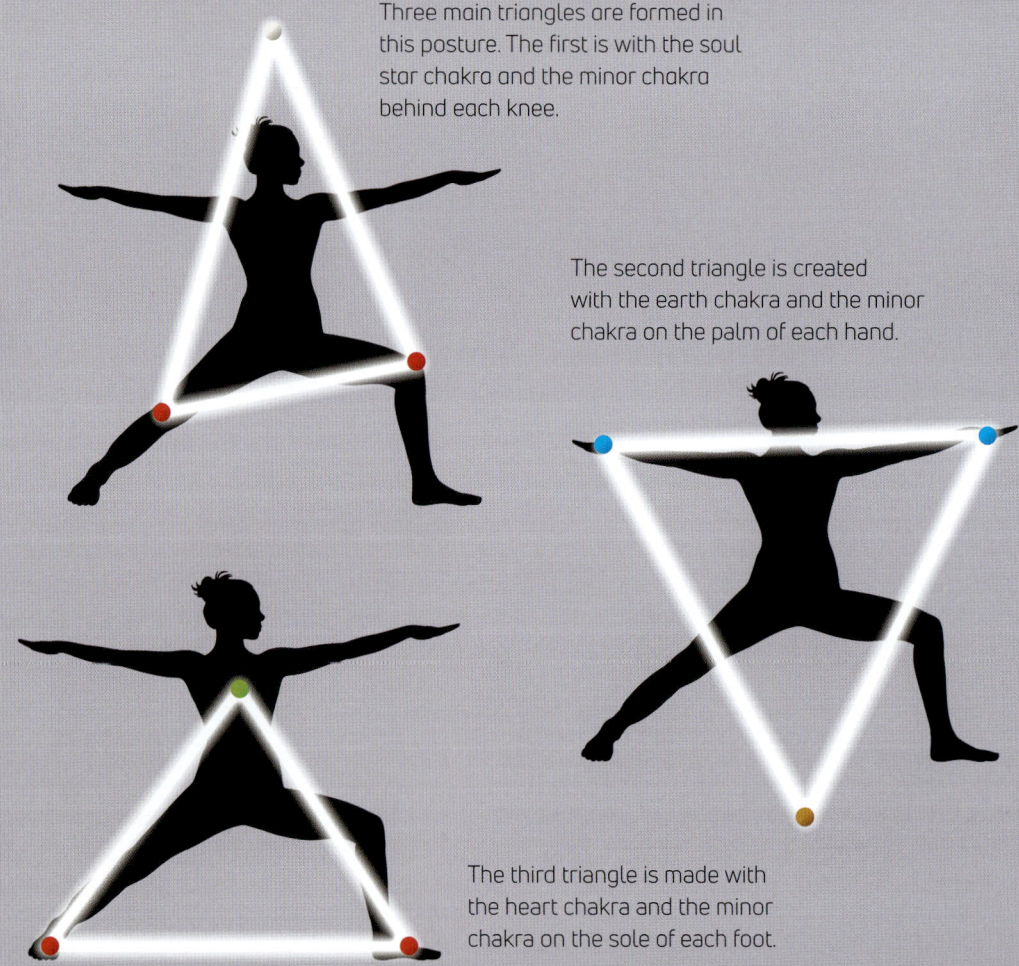

Three main triangles are formed in this posture. The first is with the soul star chakra and the minor chakra behind each knee.

The second triangle is created with the earth chakra and the minor chakra on the palm of each hand.

The third triangle is made with the heart chakra and the minor chakra on the sole of each foot.

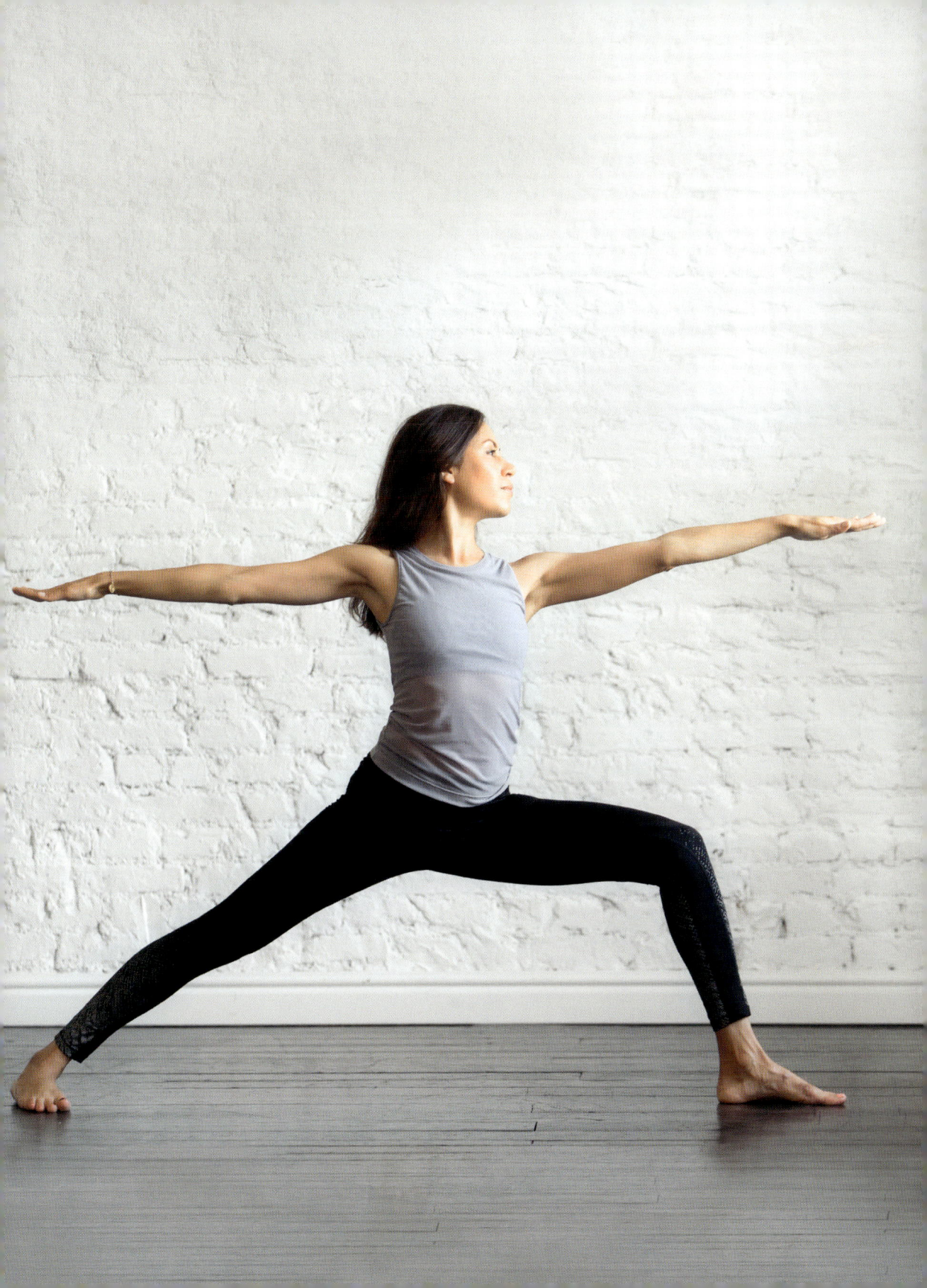

REVERSE VIRABHADRASANA
(reverse warrior posture)

Starting with the body position for warrior posture 2 (see page 122), raise your left arm up to stretch the left side of your body. Now take your right arm as far down your right leg as you can, without losing the right angle formed with the left knee. Look up to your left hand (see opposite).

   Reverse warrior posture improves the flexibility of the spine, strengthens the leg muscles, and opens the heart and the chest. The main chakra the asana works with is the heart chakra.

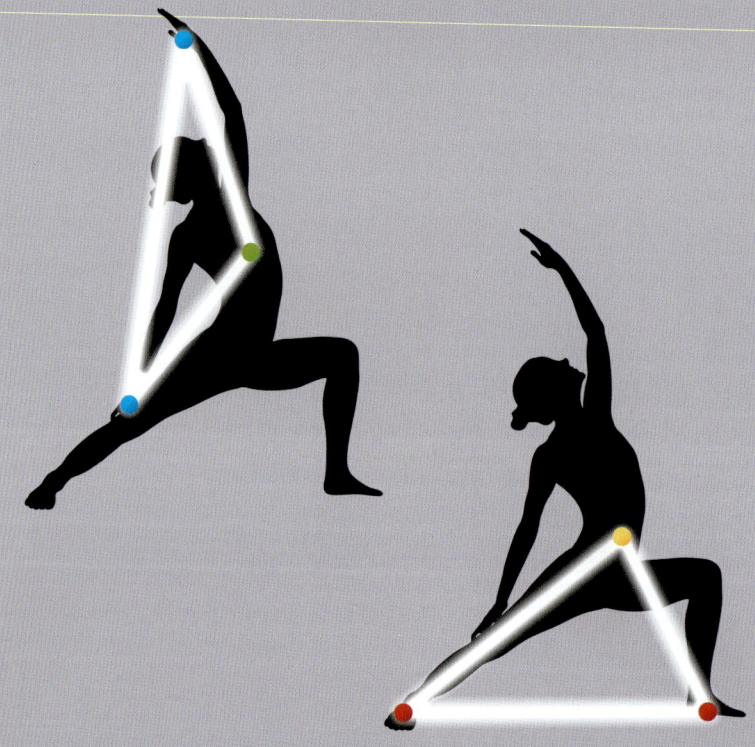

Two main triangles are formed in this posture. The first is with the heart chakra and the minor chakra on the palm of each hand. The second triangle is made with the sacral chakra and the minor chakra on the sole of each foot.

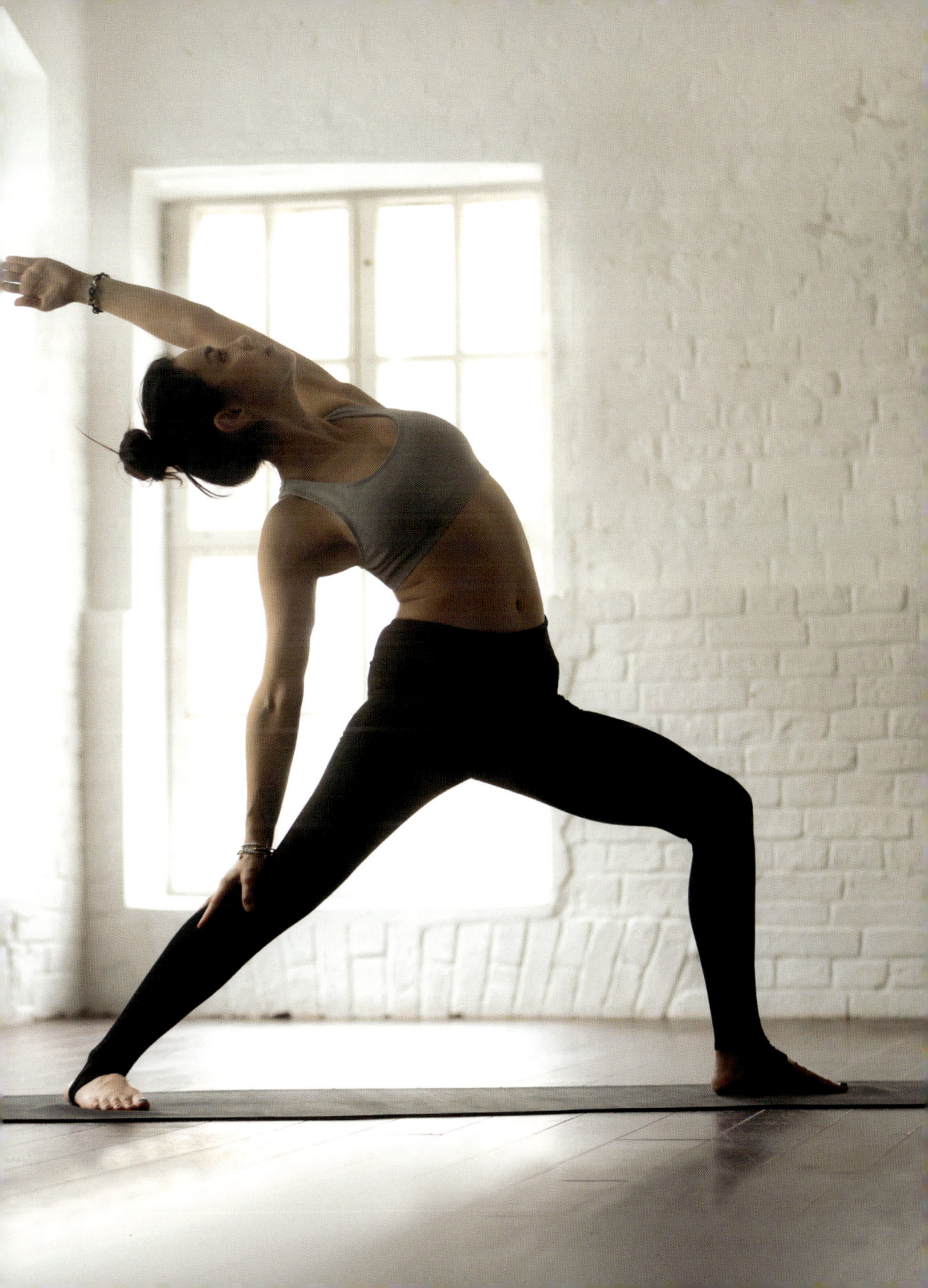

PADANGUSTHASANA (hand to foot posture)

Begin this posture in standing position, with the feet approximately 15 cm (6 in) apart, checking that your toes are in line and the feet parallel. Lift up your spine and, on the next exhalation, bend your trunk forwards from the hips, making sure that your knees are kept locked. Hold your big toes with your hands. On your next exhalation, continue to lower your trunk onto your legs, placing your hands by the side of your feet (see opposite). If you find this difficult, place books either side of your feet and place your hands on them, removing the books when your hamstring muscles become more supple. In this posture, make sure you don't lean backwards. One way of preventing this is to practise the posture standing with your back against a wall. The main chakra the asana works with is the sacral chakra.

The hand to foot posture removes excess fat around the buttocks, eliminates flatulence, constipation and indigestion, and makes the spine and back muscles supple. All the spinal nerves are stimulated and toned, and the body's metabolism is increased. The asana also works on the reproductive organs and provides a beneficial flow of blood to the brain and face.

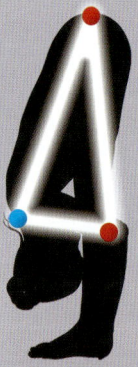

There are four main triangles of light in this posture. The first is with the base chakra, the minor chakra halfway along the clavicle bone and the minor chakra behind the knee.

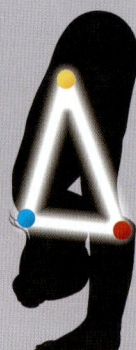

The second triangle is created with the sacral chakra, the minor chakra halfway along the clavicle bone and the minor chakra behind the knee.

The third triangle is formed with the base chakra, the earth chakra and the minor chakra midway along the clavicle bone.

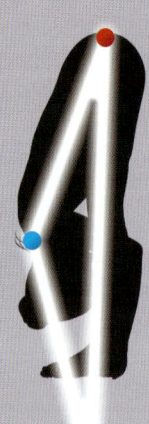

The fourth triangle is made with the minor chakras behind the knee, on the sole of the foot and behind the elbow. All four triangles appear on both sides of the body.

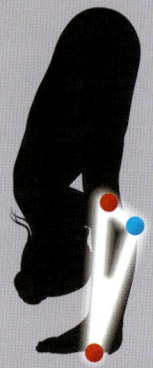

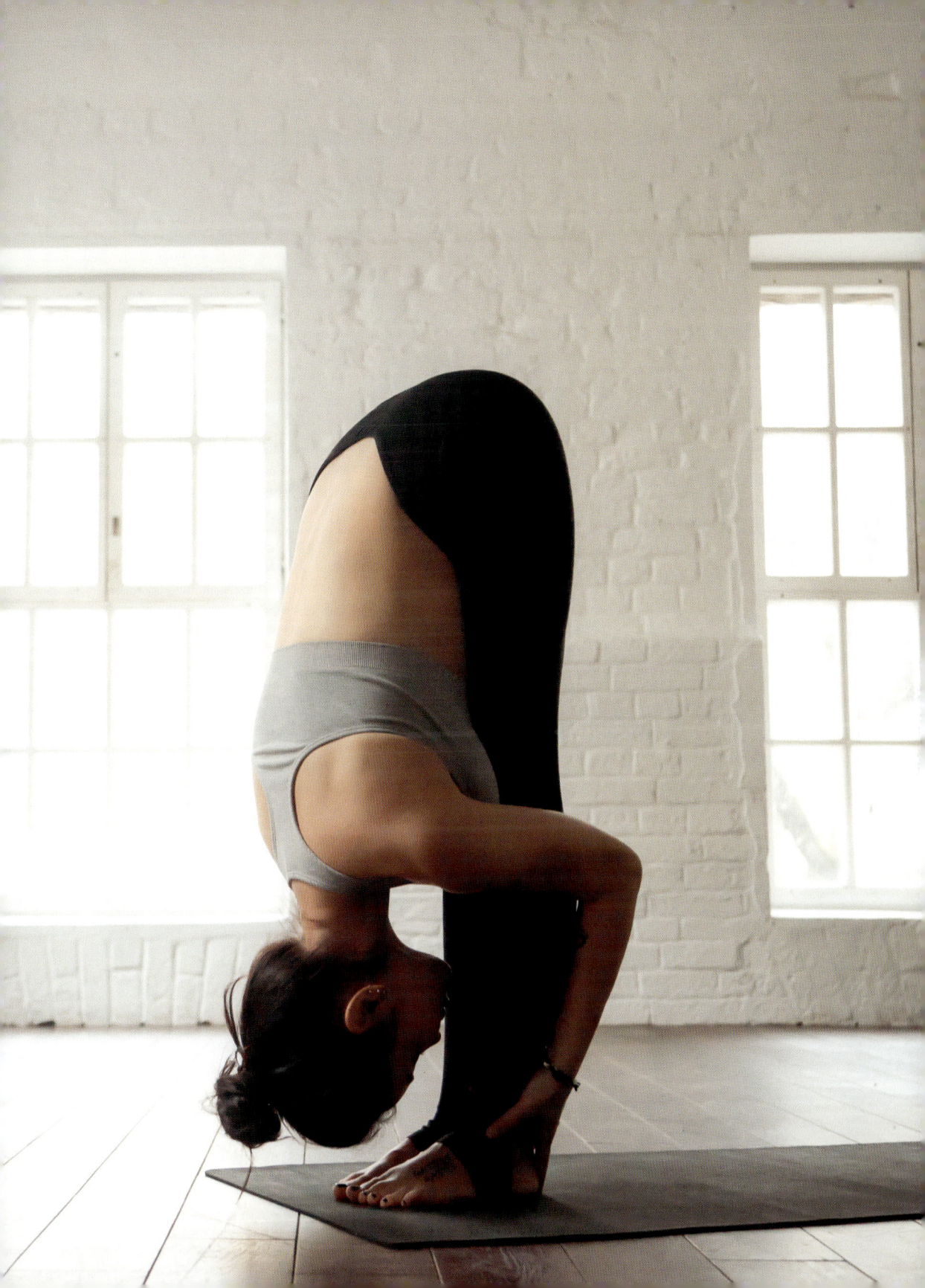

NATARAJA ASANA (Lord Shiva's posture)

Stand on the floor, with both feet together, spine straight, shoulders back and chest open. Fix your gaze on an object in front of you to help you to maintain your balance. Bend and lift your left knee and, taking your left leg behind you, hold the ankle with your left hand. Inhaling, raise your foot and leg away from your body, while raising them as high as possible. Now extend your right arm upwards and forwards, fixing your gaze on your right hand (see opposite). Make sure that the knee of the leg you're balancing on is kept locked. Hold this posture for as long as possible. Then, on an exhalation, return to the standing posture. Repeat on the opposite side. The main chakra worked with is the solar plexus chakra.

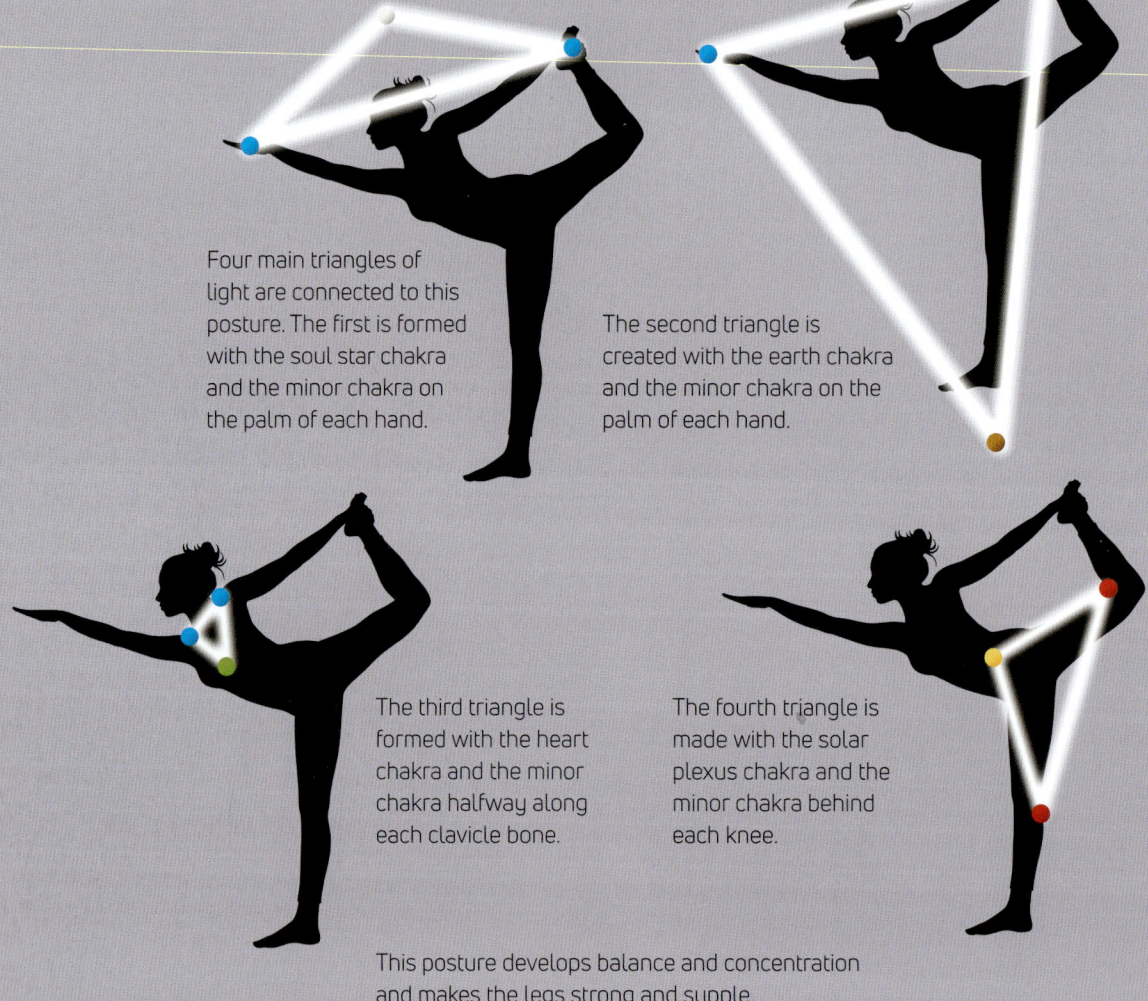

Four main triangles of light are connected to this posture. The first is formed with the soul star chakra and the minor chakra on the palm of each hand.

The second triangle is created with the earth chakra and the minor chakra on the palm of each hand.

The third triangle is formed with the heart chakra and the minor chakra halfway along each clavicle bone.

The fourth triangle is made with the solar plexus chakra and the minor chakra behind each knee.

This posture develops balance and concentration and makes the legs strong and supple.

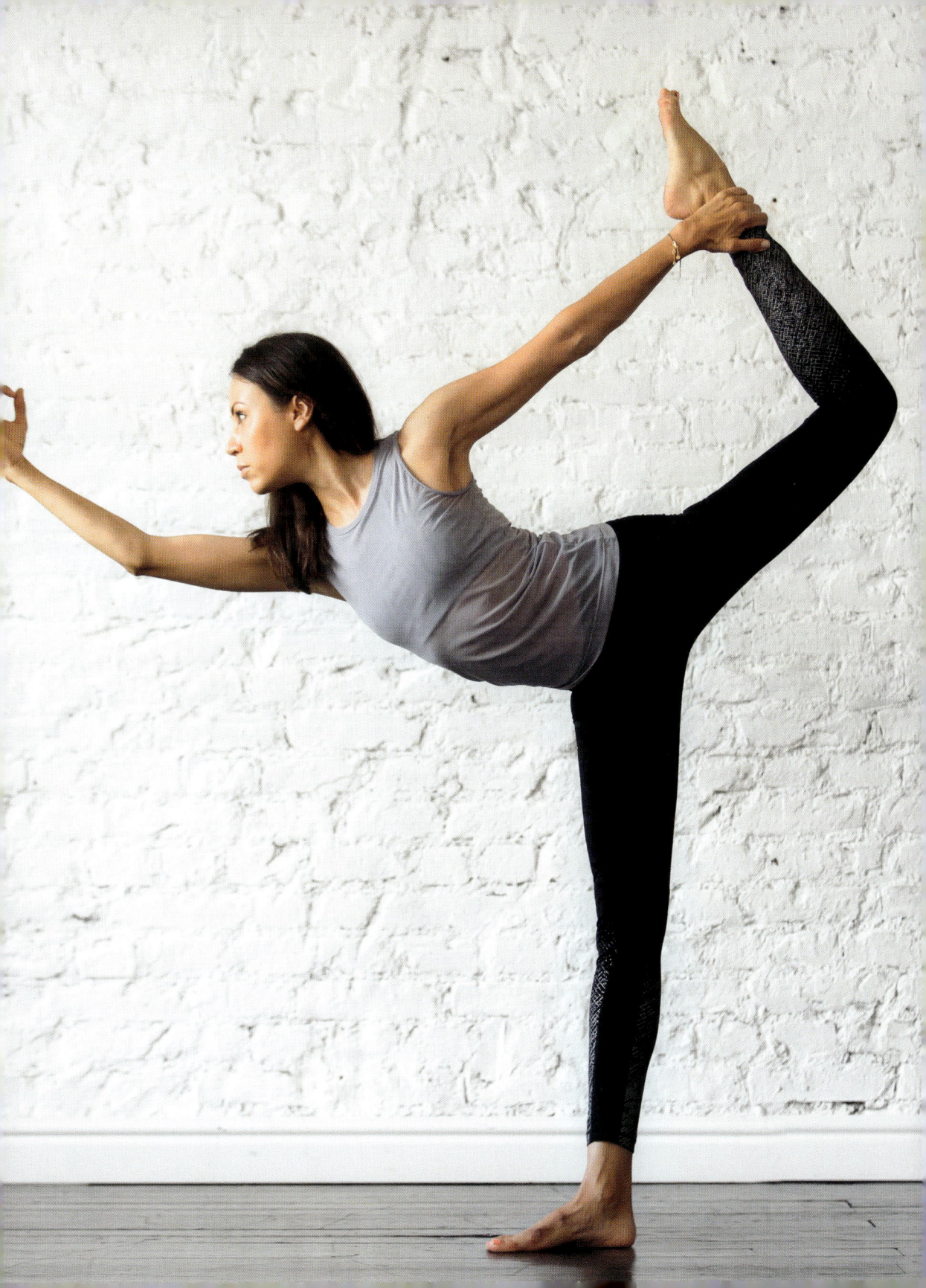

ARDHA CHANDRASANA
(half-moon posture)

The half-moon is a balance posture, but you can use a wall for support. Standing against a wall, bring your right hand down onto a yoga brick or some books. With your right leg kept straight and your knee locked, raise your left leg, forming a straight line along the left side of your body. Raise your left arm, bringing it in line with your right arm. Look up towards your left hand. Repeat on the opposite side.

The posture strengthens the back, thighs, ankles, abdomen and the lumbar and sacrum spine. When it's done free-standing (see opposite), it creates a sense of balance and stability. With the chest fully open, the heart chakra is activated.

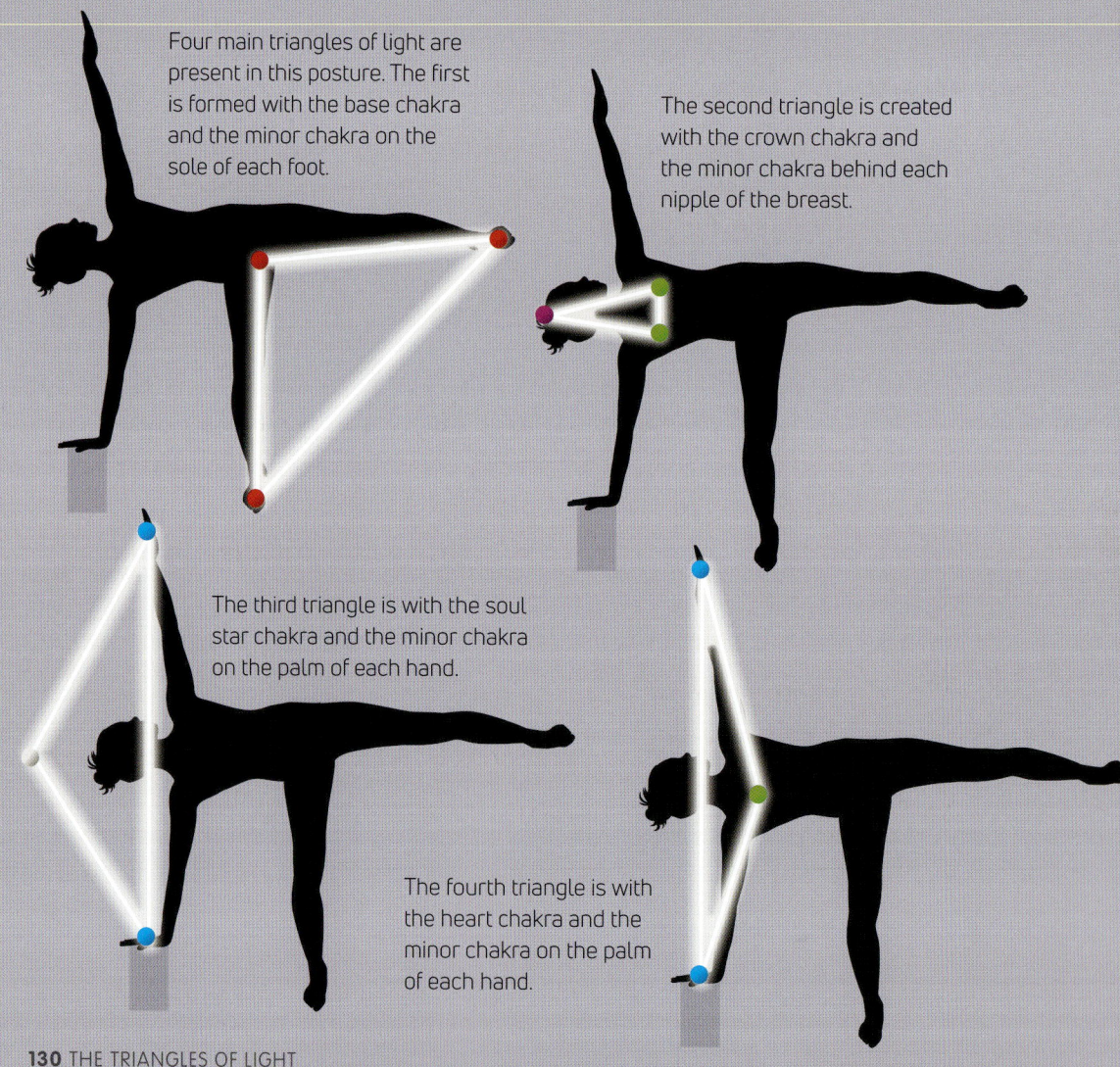

Four main triangles of light are present in this posture. The first is formed with the base chakra and the minor chakra on the sole of each foot.

The second triangle is created with the crown chakra and the minor chakra behind each nipple of the breast.

The third triangle is with the soul star chakra and the minor chakra on the palm of each hand.

The fourth triangle is with the heart chakra and the minor chakra on the palm of each hand.

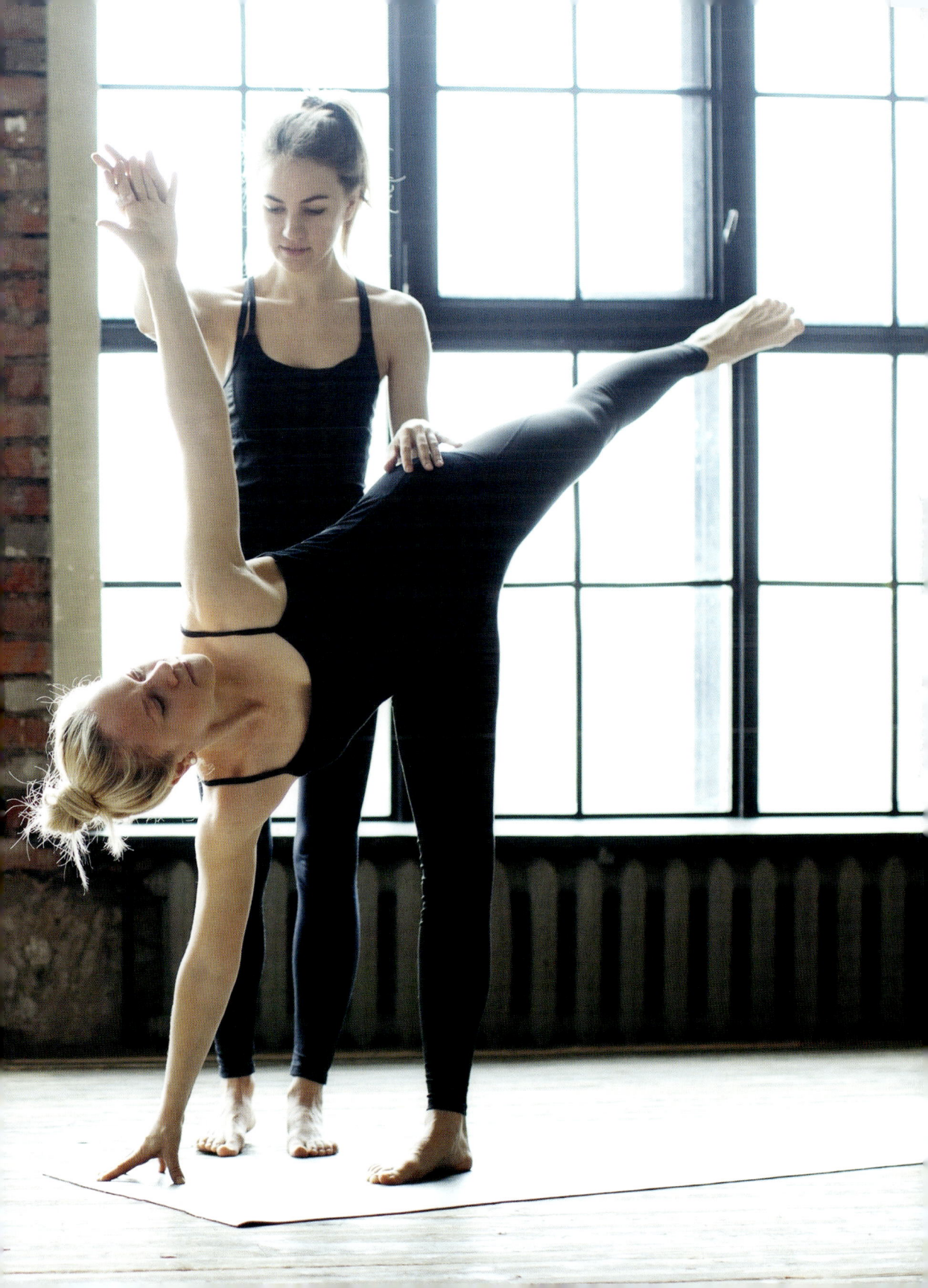

SUPTA VIRASANA (reclined hero posture)

Kneel on the floor with your legs and feet together, and sit back on your feet. Slide your feet outwards a little, so that they are alongside your buttocks, and, exhaling, bend your trunk backwards, supporting your body on your arms and elbows until the top of your head touches the floor with your back fully arched. Now take your arms off the floor, placing your hands on your thighs and making sure that your knees stay together on the ground. Hold this posture for as long as is comfortable. If you find this posture difficult, separate your knees until your thigh muscles and spine become supple enough to allow the knees to be brought together. Alternatively, place a blanket or blankets under your head.

The reclined hero posture works with the abdomen and is beneficial for those suffering from constipation. It tones the spinal nerves and benefits the thyroid and parathyroid glands. It also tones the thigh muscles and helps to strengthen the knees. The main chakra the asana works with is the throat chakra.

Three major triangles of light are activated in this posture. The first is with the throat chakra and the minor chakra on the palm of each hand.

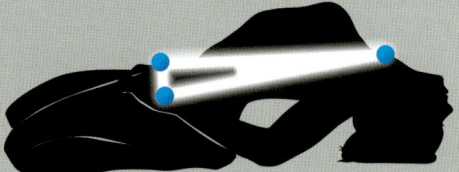

The second triangle is formed with the heart chakra, the crown chakra and the minor chakra on the sole of the foot. This triangle appears on both sides of the body.

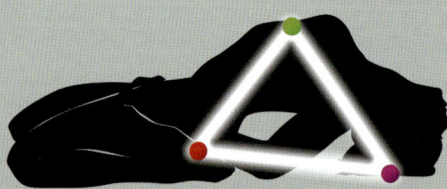

The third triangle is created with the solar plexus chakra and the minor chakra behind each knee.

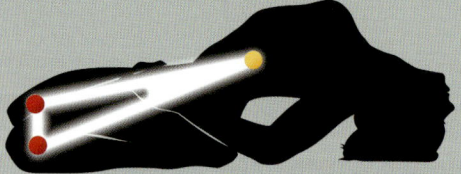

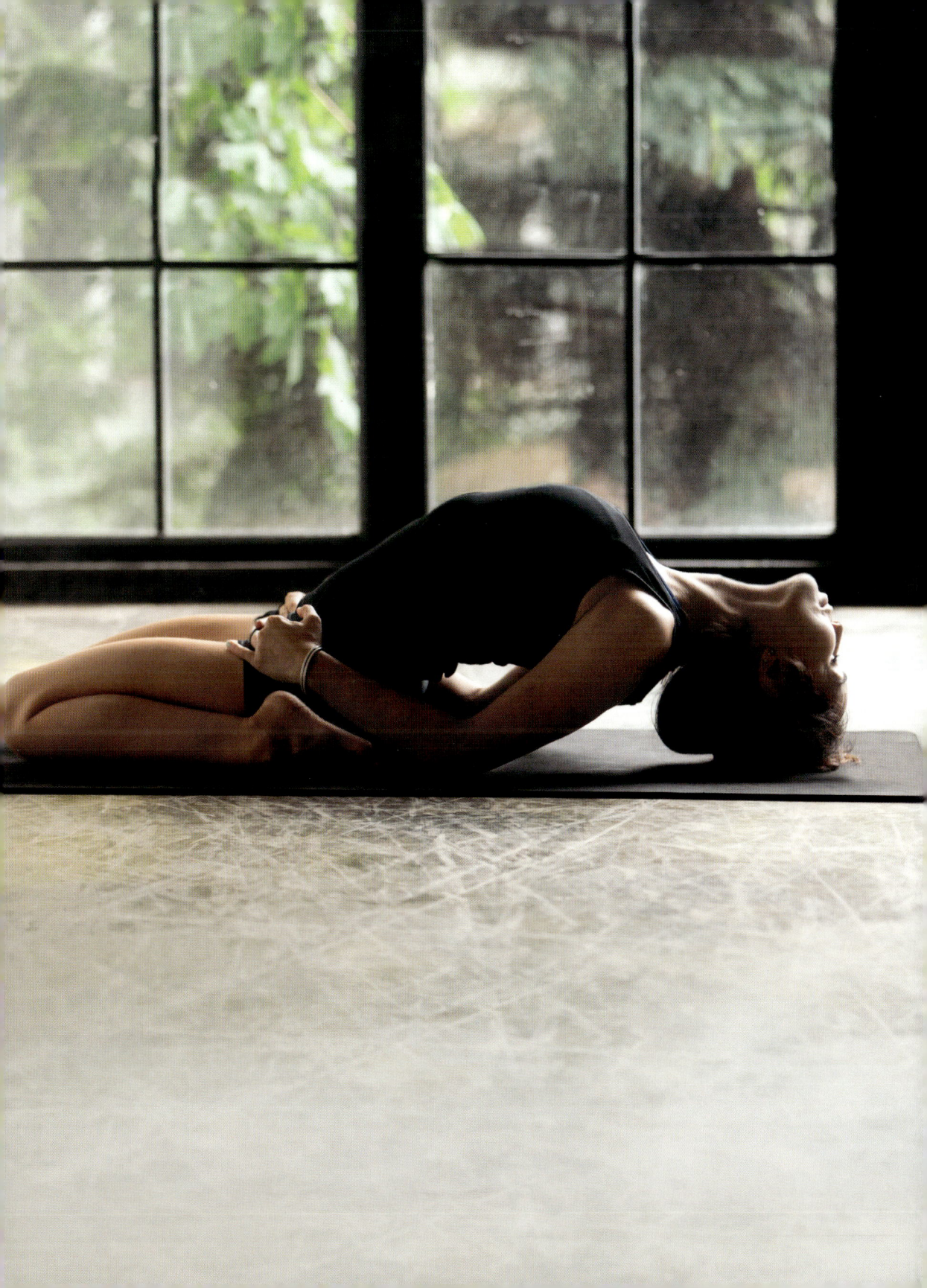

SALABHASANA (locust posture)

Lie on your stomach, with your chin resting on the floor and your hands clasped underneath your thighs with both your thumbs on the floor. Stretch your legs and tense your arms. Inhale, and, holding your breath in, raise your legs and abdomen as high off the ground as possible, at the same time raising your head and shoulders off the ground (keeping your chest on the floor, as shown here). Then, on an exhalation, lower your legs back onto the floor. If you wish to try a more advanced version of this posture (known as 'inverted locust'), keep your chin resting on the floor when you raise your legs

This asana tones the liver and other abdominal organs, especially the pancreas, intestines and kidneys. The bladder and prostate gland also benefit. The posture stimulates the appetite and relieves any stomach problems. It also strengthens the lower spine and abdominal muscles and tones the sciatic nerve. The main chakra activated is the solar plexus chakra.

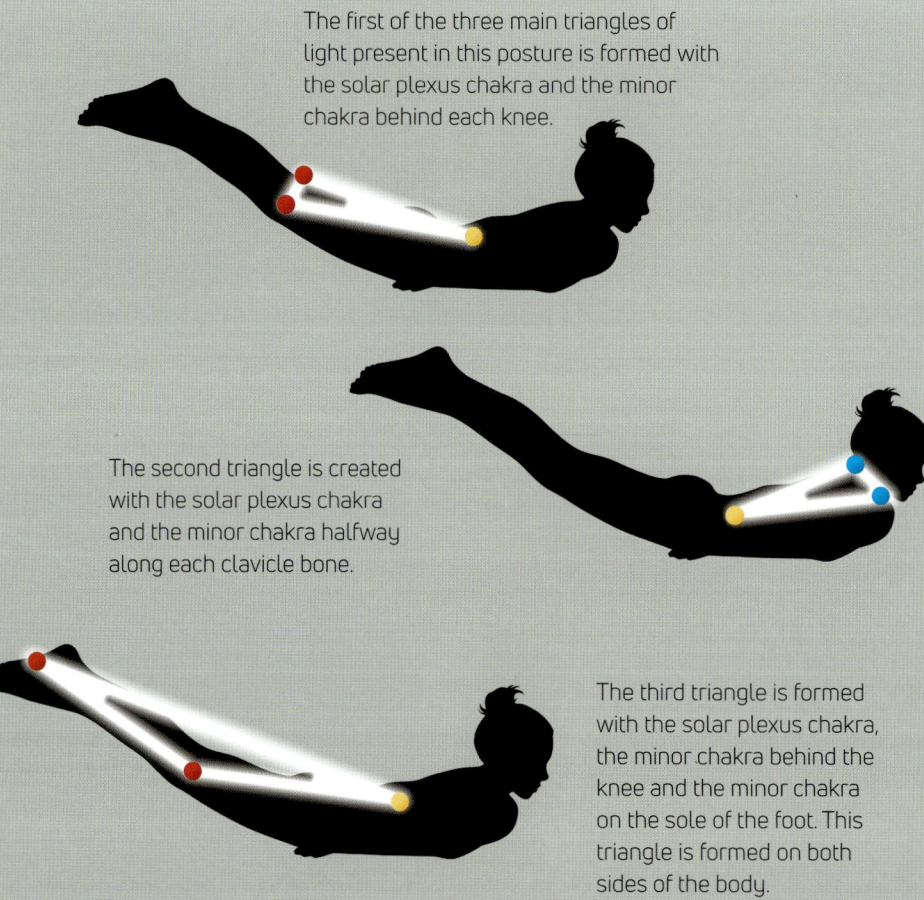

The first of the three main triangles of light present in this posture is formed with the solar plexus chakra and the minor chakra behind each knee.

The second triangle is created with the solar plexus chakra and the minor chakra halfway along each clavicle bone.

The third triangle is formed with the solar plexus chakra, the minor chakra behind the knee and the minor chakra on the sole of the foot. This triangle is formed on both sides of the body.

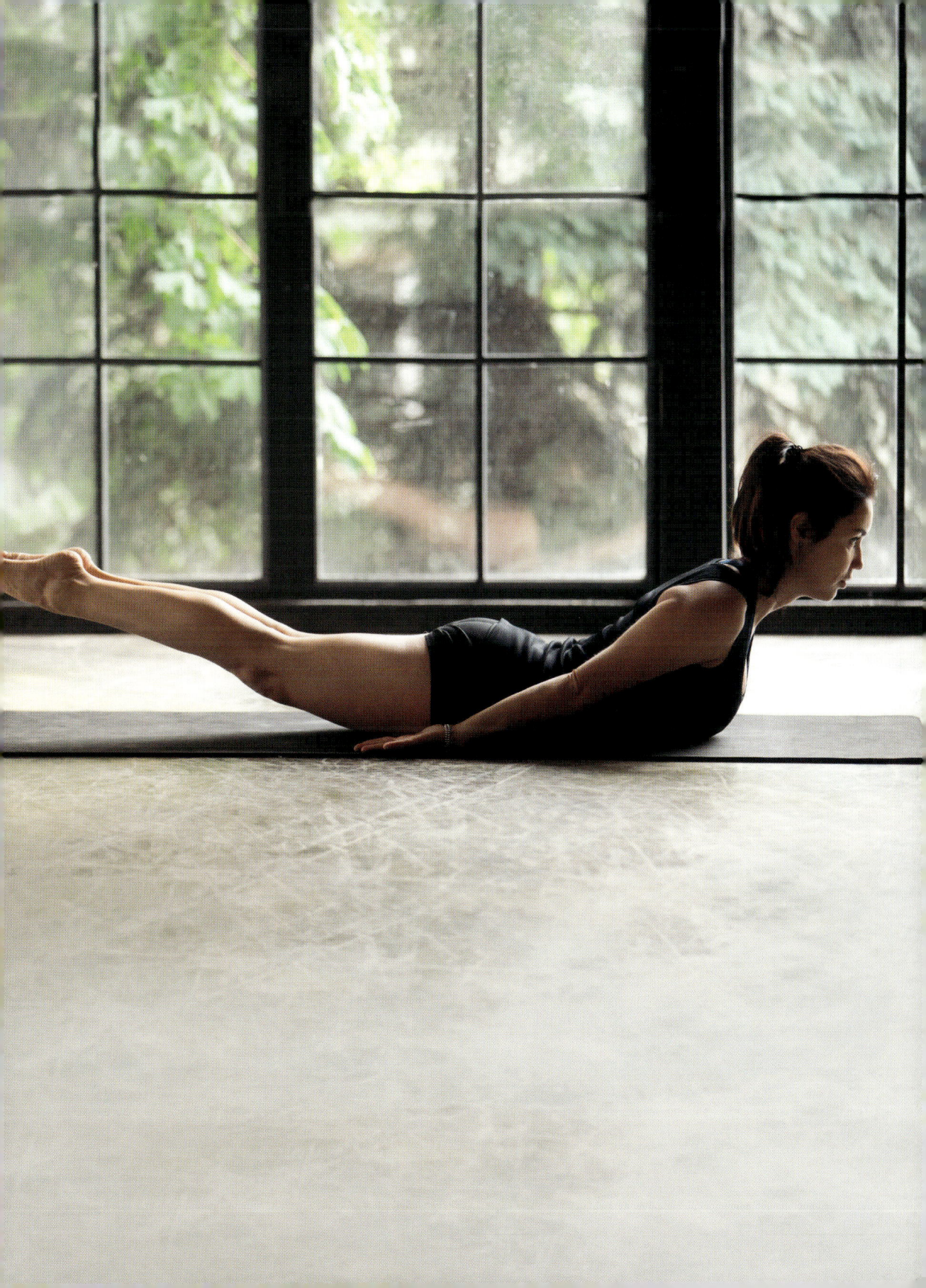

USTRASANA (camel posture)

Kneel on the floor, with your knees and feet together. Exhale, and place your right hand on your right heel and your left hand on your left heel. If you find this difficult, either tuck your toes under or place folded blankets on your legs as support for your hands. Pressing down with your hands, and taking your head back, push your trunk up until your thighs are in line with your knees (see opposite). A good way to practise this posture is against a wall. Facing the wall, push your trunk up until your abdomen and thighs touch the wall. Hold this posture for as long as is comfortable, then release your hands and sit back on your heels. The main chakra worked with ustrasana is the solar plexus chakra.

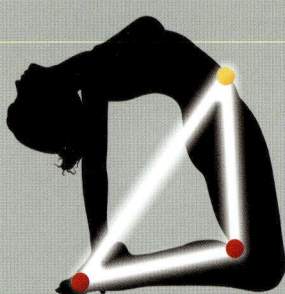

The first triangle of light formed in this posture is between the solar plexus chakra, the minor chakra behind the knee and the minor chakra on the sole of the foot.

The second triangle is created with the solar plexus chakra, the throat chakra and the minor chakra on the palm of the hand. The first and second triangles of light are formed on both sides of the body.

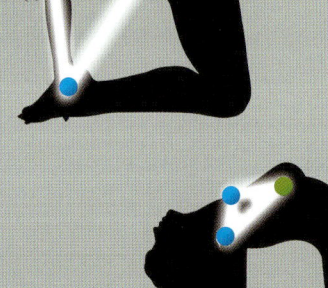

The third triangle is formed with the heart chakra and the minor chakra found halfway along each clavicle bone.

The camel posture stretches and tones the whole of the spine, making it supple. It also works on the abdominal muscles and on the shoulder joints.

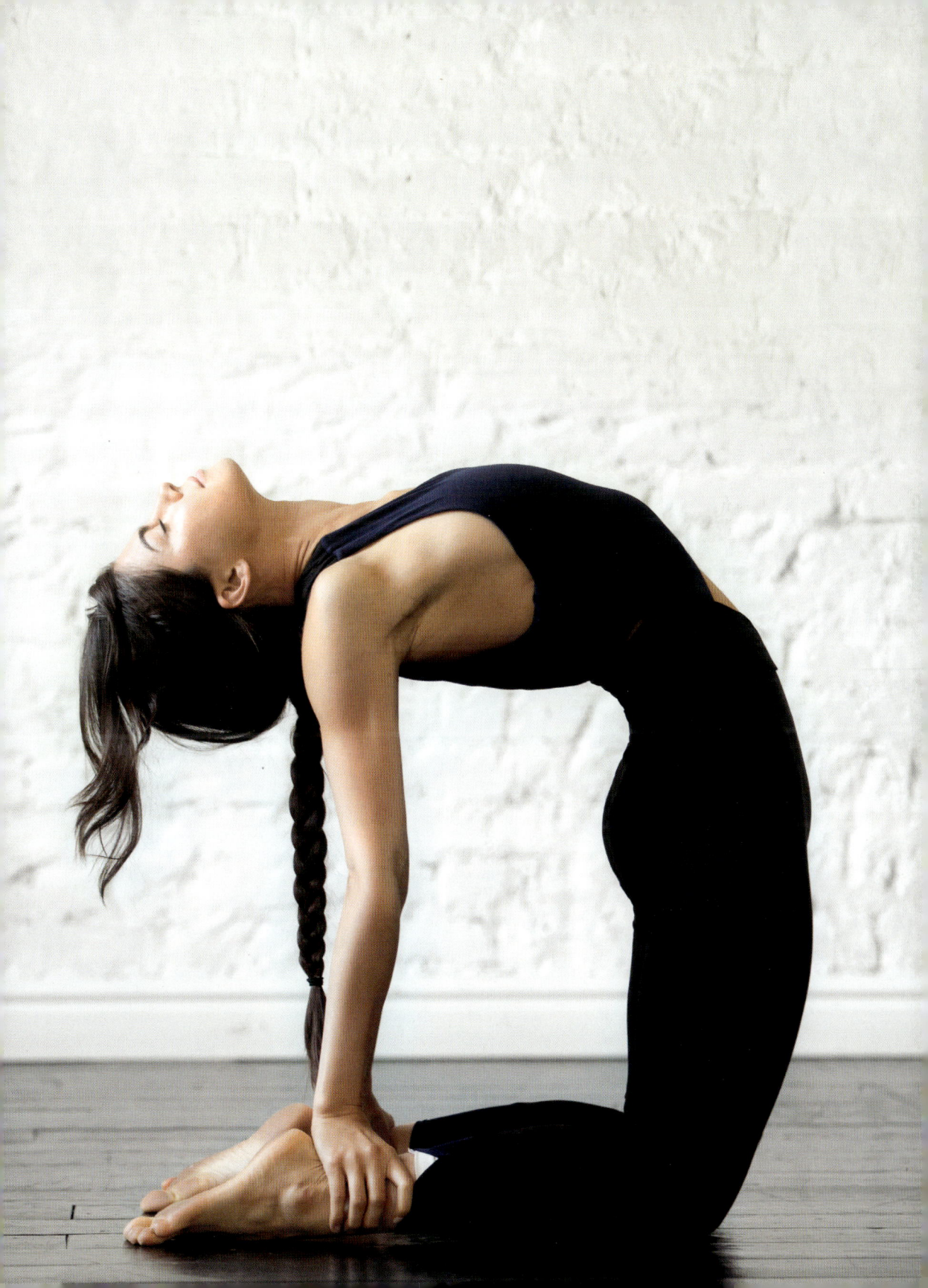

BHUJANGASANA ASANA (cobra posture)

Lie flat on the floor, with your chin resting on the floor. Place your hands by your chest, with fingers pointing towards the head. Inhale, and lift your trunk off the floor, keeping your abdomen in contact with the floor and legs straight. Take your shoulders down and back, keeping your head in line with your spine (see opposite). Hold the posture for as long as is comfortable, then, exhaling, bend your elbows and return to the start position. If your spine is stiff, work with your legs apart, or start by working with your elbows and hands on the floor; this is known as the sphinx posture, which works with the solar plexus chakra.

The cobra posture rejuvenates the spine, relieves stiff back muscles and sciatica, and works with female disorders such as vaginal discharge, painful menstruation and missed periods. It also benefits the kidneys and bladder, tones the uterus and ovaries, alleviates water retention, stimulates the appetite and helps to eliminate constipation.

There are three main triangles of light present in this asana. The first is between the soul star chakra, the heart chakra and the solar plexus chakra.

The second triangle is formed with the sacral chakra and the minor chakra on the palm of each hand.

The third triangle – present on both sides of the body – is created with the minor chakra on the sole of the foot, the minor chakra halfway along the clavicle bone and the minor chakra on the palm of the hand.

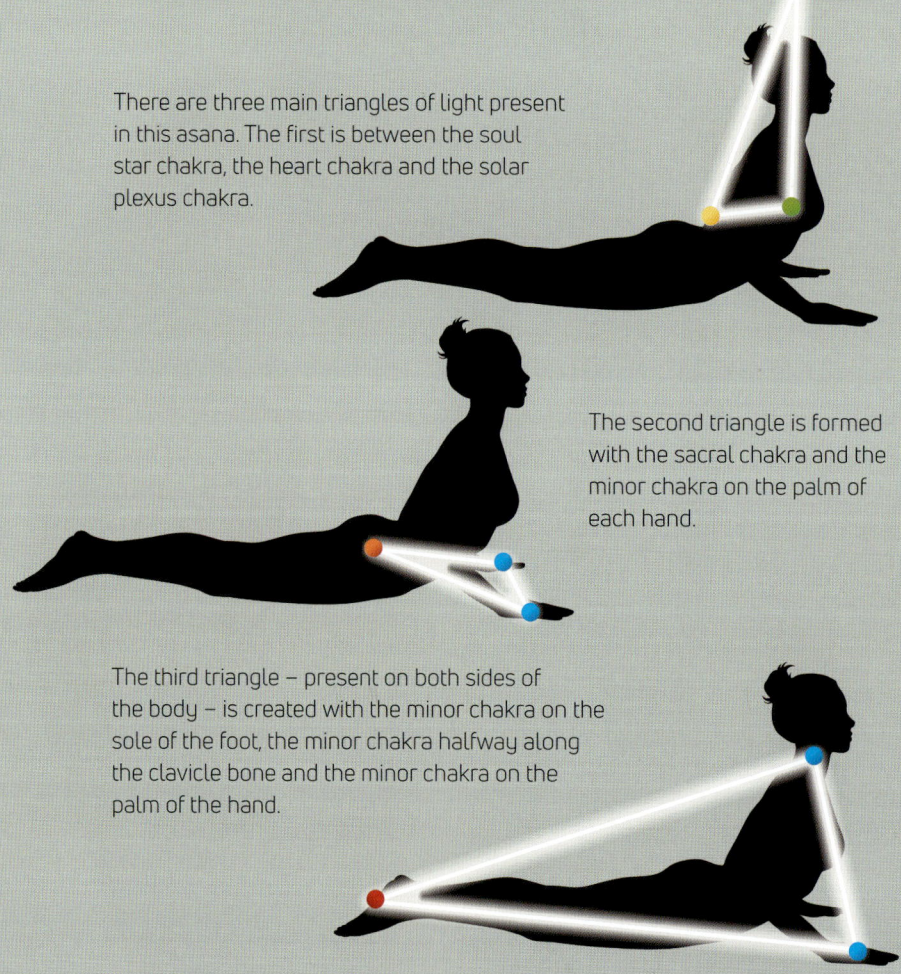

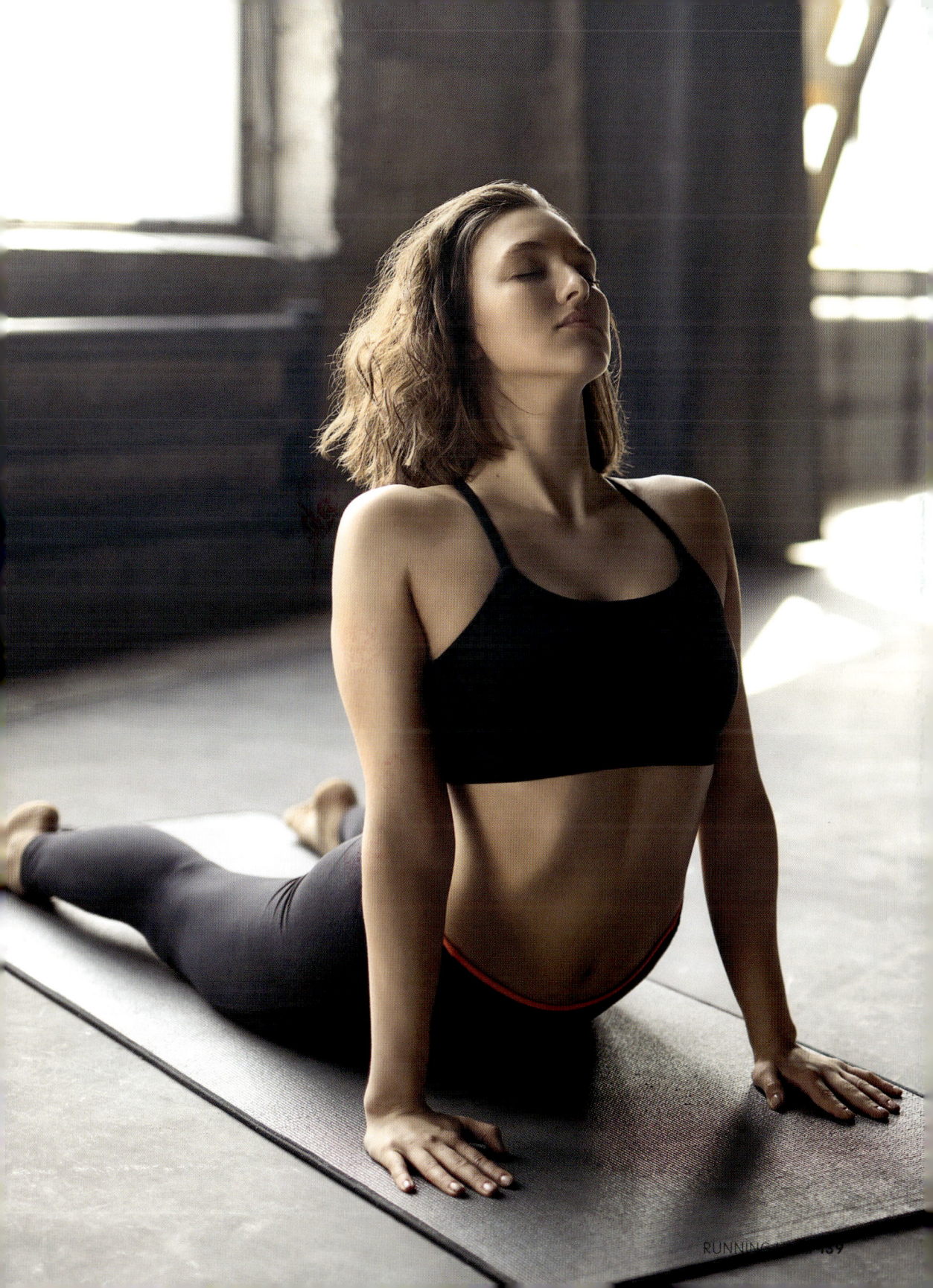

DHANURASANA (bow posture)

Lie on the floor, face downwards. Bend your knees and hold your ankles with your hands. This is the intermediate position. Exhaling, raise your legs and chest off the floor (see opposite). Lift your head and take it as far back as possible. If you can't raise your legs, gently work with the intermediate position until you're able to go into the full posture.

Dhanurasana works on the abdominal muscles and hips. It tones the muscles of the back, makes the spine flexible and reduces abdominal fat. The chakra worked with is the solar plexus chakra.

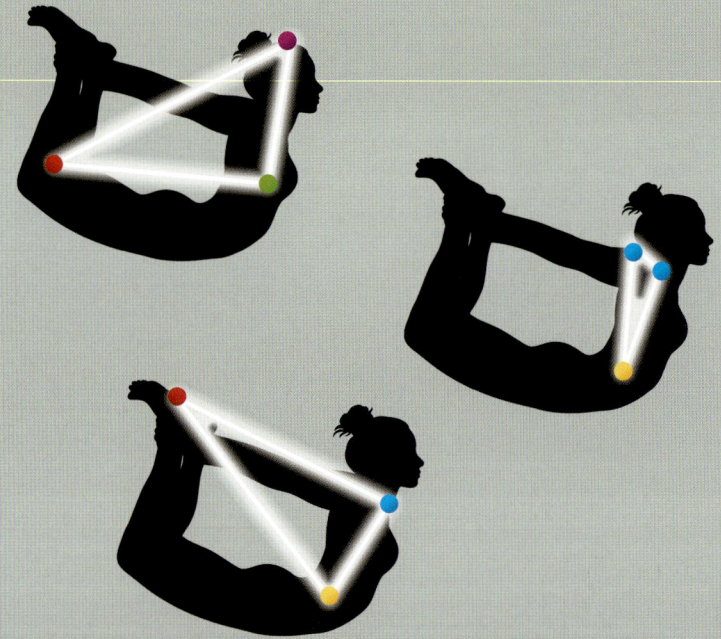

There are three main triangles of light formed in this posture. The first – present on both sides of the body – is with the crown chakra, the heart chakra and the minor chakra behind the knee. The second triangle is created with the solar plexus chakra and the minor chakra halfway along each clavicle bone. The third triangle – also present on both sides of the body – is made with the solar plexus chakra, the throat chakra and the minor chakra on the sole of the foot.

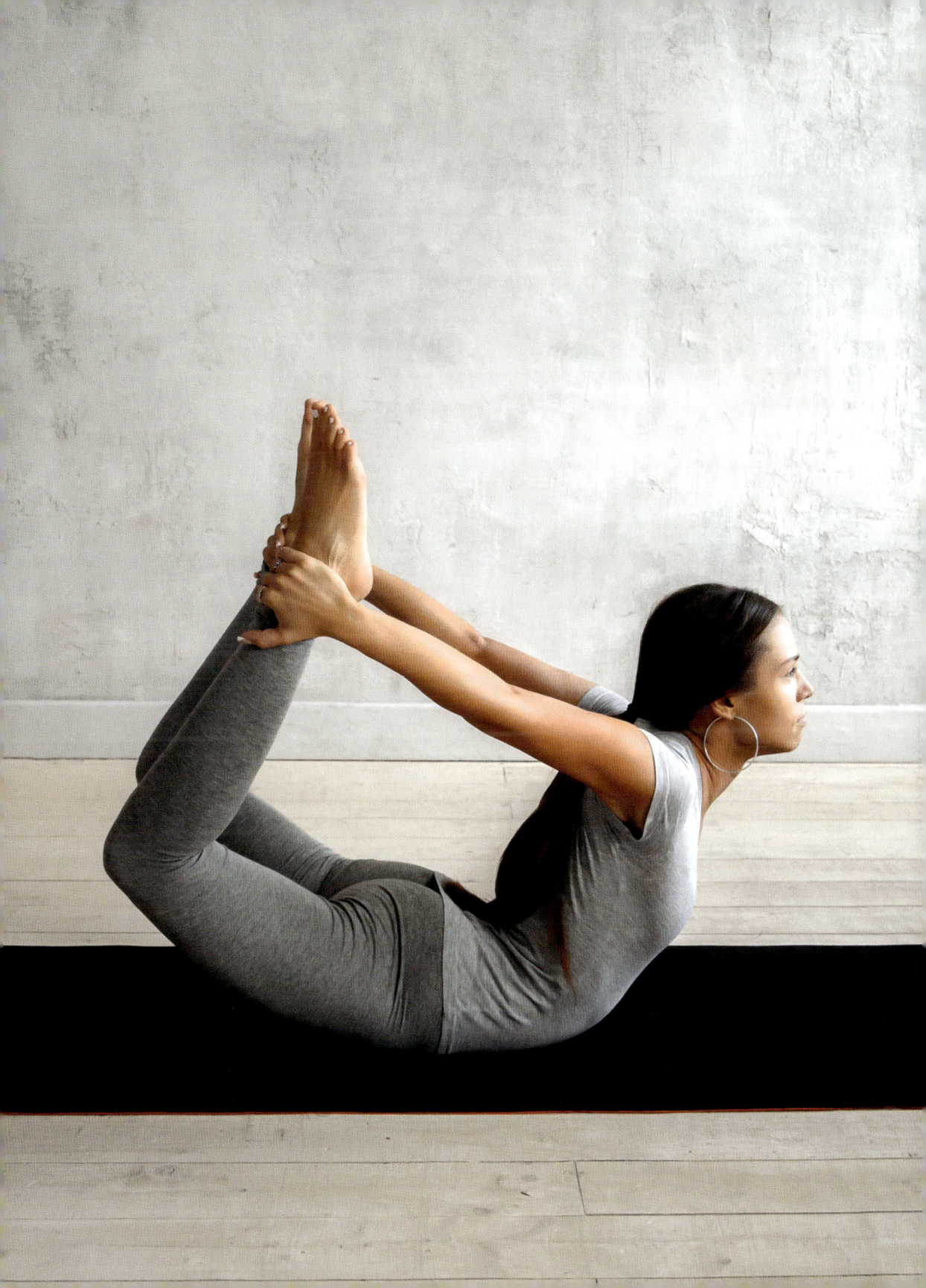

UTTANA MAYURASANA (bridge posture)

Lie flat on the floor. Bend your knees and place the soles of your feet by your buttocks. On your next inhalation, press down with your feet and raise your trunk off the floor, supporting your back with the palms of your hands (see opposite). Make sure that your hands and elbows are in a straight line. Keep your shoulders on the floor, with your neck extended and knees held together. Hold for as long as is comfortable, before lowering your body back onto the floor. If you find this posture difficult, you can use a wooden yoga block, placing this beneath your buttocks and laying your arms on the floor by the side of your raised body. Continue to use the wooden block until you're able to support your body on your hands and arms.

Three main triangles – all present on both sides of the body – are formed in this posture. The first is with the soul star chakra, the earth chakra and the minor chakra behind the knee.

The second triangle is created with the throat chakra, the solar plexus chakra and the minor chakra in the crease of the elbow.

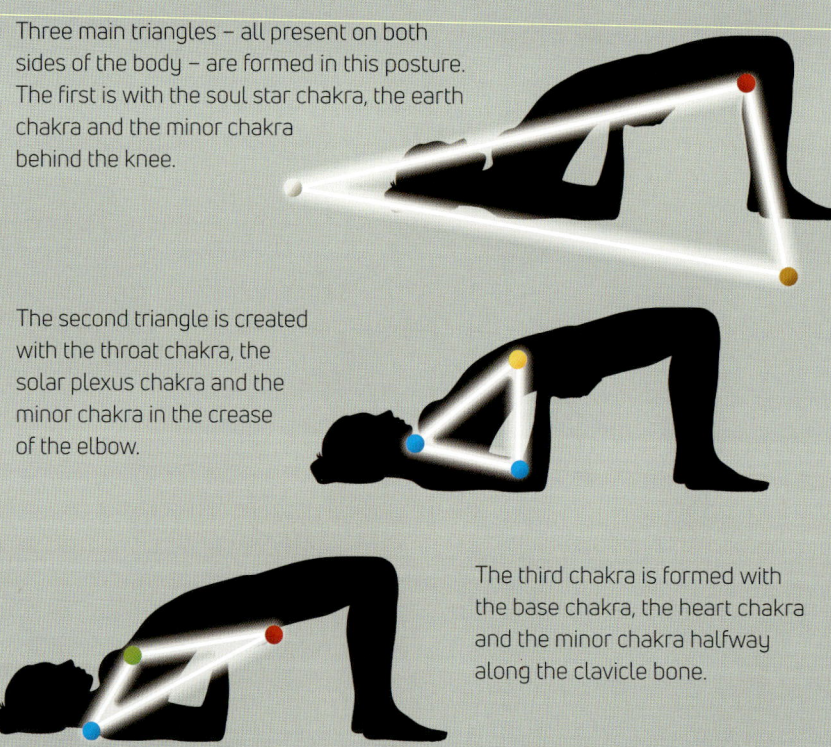

The third chakra is formed with the base chakra, the heart chakra and the minor chakra halfway along the clavicle bone.

This posture strengthens and makes supple the back and wrist joints. It also tones the abdominal organs and works on the thigh muscles. The two main chakras worked with are the throat chakra and the solar plexus chakra.

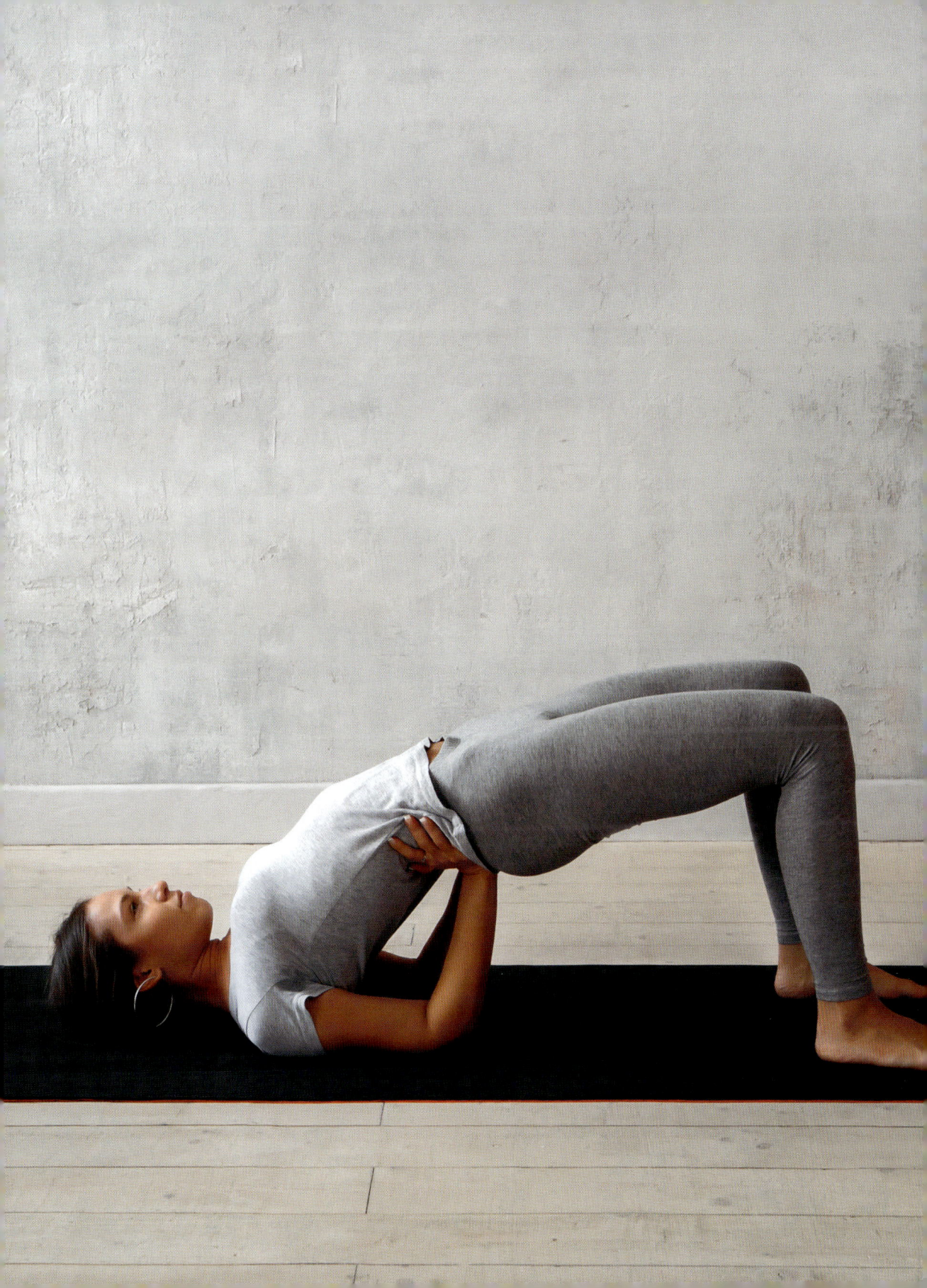

URDHVA DHANURASANA (wheel posture)

The wheel is an advanced posture. Before attempting it, you should work first with the bridge posture (see page 142) to make your spine more supple.

Lie flat on the floor, bend your elbows and take your arms over your head, placing the palms of your hands under your shoulders with your fingers pointing towards your feet. Bend your knees, placing the soles of your feet by your buttocks. On your next exhalation, push down with your hands and feet to raise the trunk off the floor, allowing your head to rest on the floor. This is the intermediate position. Now press down again with your hands and feet to straighten the arms and lift the head off the floor (see opposite). Hold for as long as is comfortable.

This posture benefits the entire nervous system and hormonal glands, and can relieve various ailments connected with the female reproductive system. It also helps to make the back muscles more supple and powerfully compresses and massages the abdominal organs. The wheel works with all seven chakras.

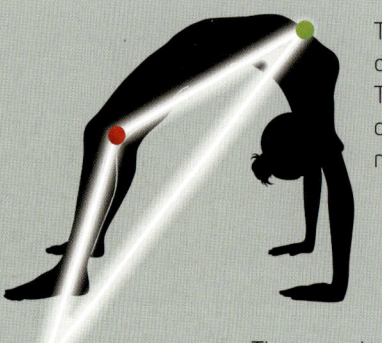

There are three main triangles of light in the wheel posture. The first is formed with the heart chakra, the earth chakra and the minor chakra behind the knee.

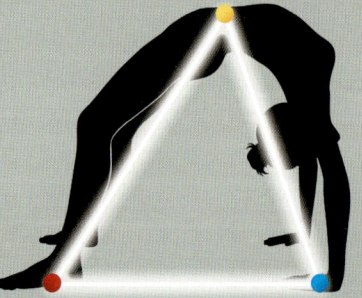

The second triangle is created with the solar plexus chakra, the minor chakra on the sole of the foot and the minor chakra on the palm of the hand.

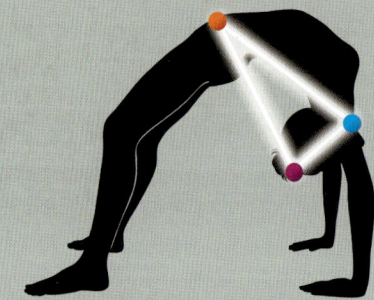

The third triangle is formed with the crown chakra, the sacral chakra and the throat chakra. All three triangles are formed on both sides of the body.

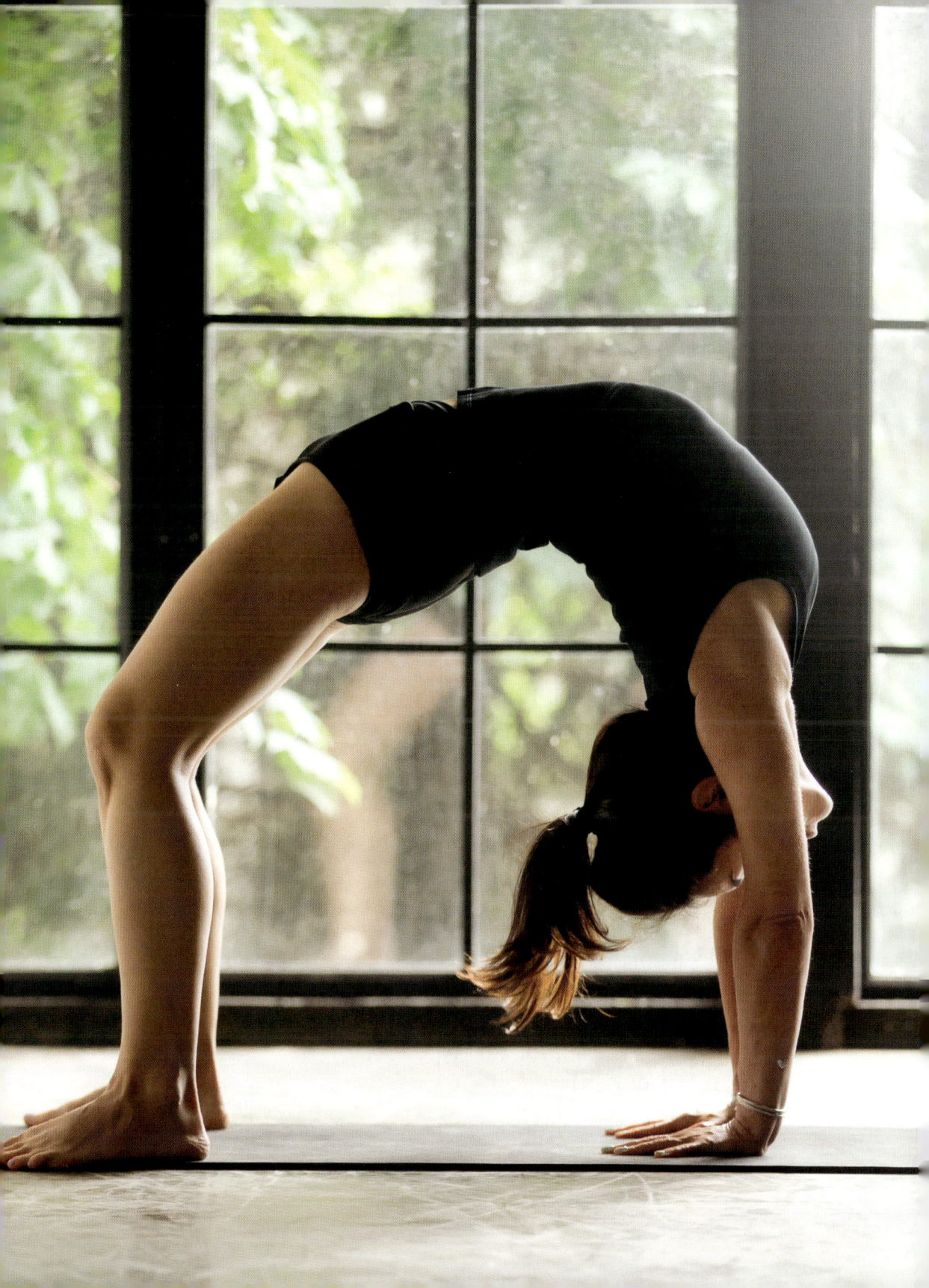

BAKASANA (crane posture)

Kneel on the floor. Place your hands on the floor, beneath your shoulders and in line with your knees. Place the crown of your head on the floor, approximately 15 cm (6 in) in front of your hands, making a triangle with the head and hands. Straighten your legs, and then walk your feet towards your hands until your spine is straight. Bend your left knee and place this on your left elbow. Now bend your right knee and place this on your right elbow. Bring both your feet together to form the tail of the bird (see opposite). Hold for as long as possible, before coming out of the posture and relaxing. If you find it difficult to balance, bakasana can be done with your back against a wall.

This posture helps you to gain a sense of balance and is also a good asana to try before the headstand (see page 148). It strengthens the arms and wrists and gives the head a fresh supply of blood. The crane works with the crown chakra.

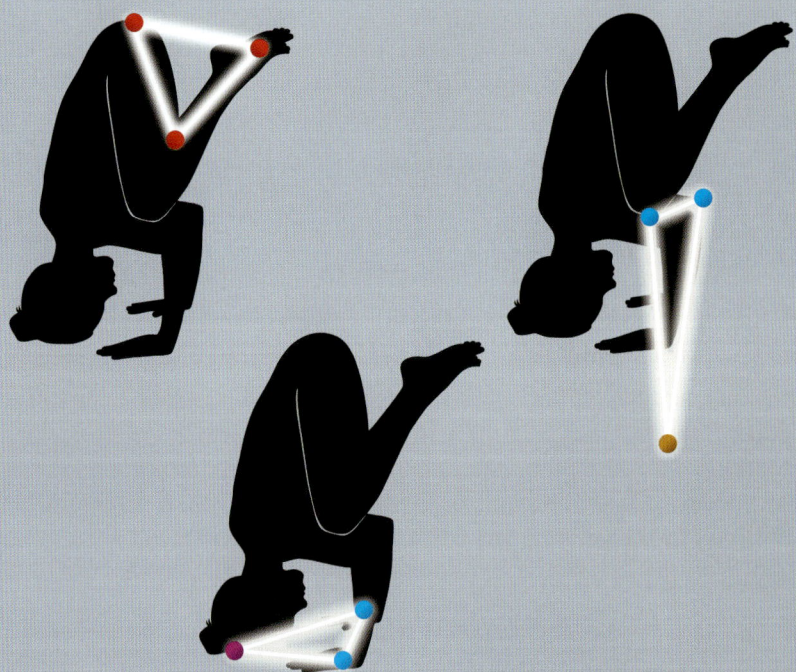

Three main triangles of light are formed with this posture. The first – present on both sides of the body – is with the base chakra, the minor chakra behind the knee and the minor chakra on the sole of the foot. The second triangle is created with the earth chakra and the minor chakra in the crease of each elbow. The third triangle is made with the crown chakra and the minor chakra on the palm of each hand.

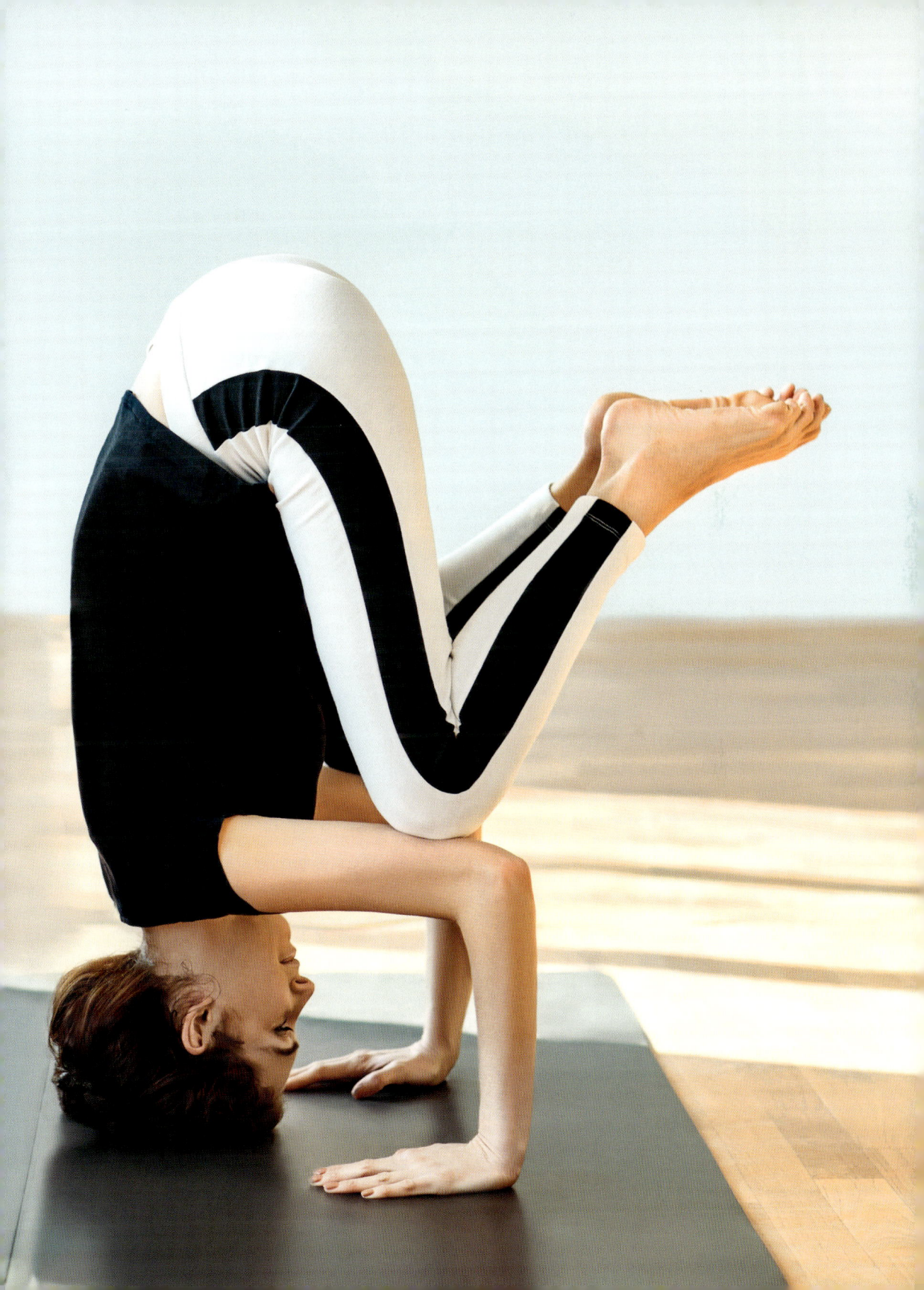

SIRSASANA (headstand)

You should practise this asana against a wall until you have gained your balance and confidence. Fold a blanket, or work with your yoga mat, and place this on the floor in front of your body and close to the wall. Kneel on the floor in front of the blanket. Clasp your hands and, bending your elbows, place them on the blanket. Make sure that your lower arms are parallel and elbows in line with your shoulders. Place the crown of your head on the blanket, between your cupped hands, allowing the back of your head to touch the palms of your hands. Straighten your legs, bringing your feet onto the floor. Slowly walk your feet towards your head until your thighs come into contact with your abdomen. Lift up your spine and gradually take the balance and weight of your body on your arms and head (see opposite). Now slowly take one leg off the floor and place it against the wall – then do the same with your other leg. When you're in the headstand, press down with your arms to straighten the spine and to take the pressure off your head and cervical spine. To begin with, try to hold this posture for 30 seconds. Then, gradually and with practice, increase the time to 20 minutes. When you're ready to come out of the posture, bend your knees and place your feet on the wall before lowering your legs back down to the floor. Go into child's pose (see below) and relax (if you try to stand or sit up straight away, the blood that has concentrated in your head and neck will suddenly drain into the rest of the body, which can leave you feeling dizzy).

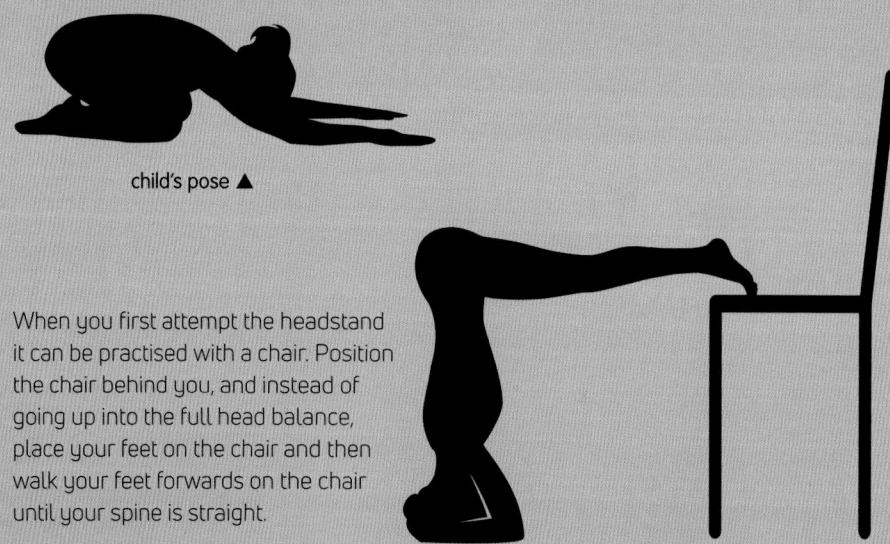

child's pose ▲

When you first attempt the headstand it can be practised with a chair. Position the chair behind you, and instead of going up into the full head balance, place your feet on the chair and then walk your feet forwards on the chair until your spine is straight.

continued overleaf ▶

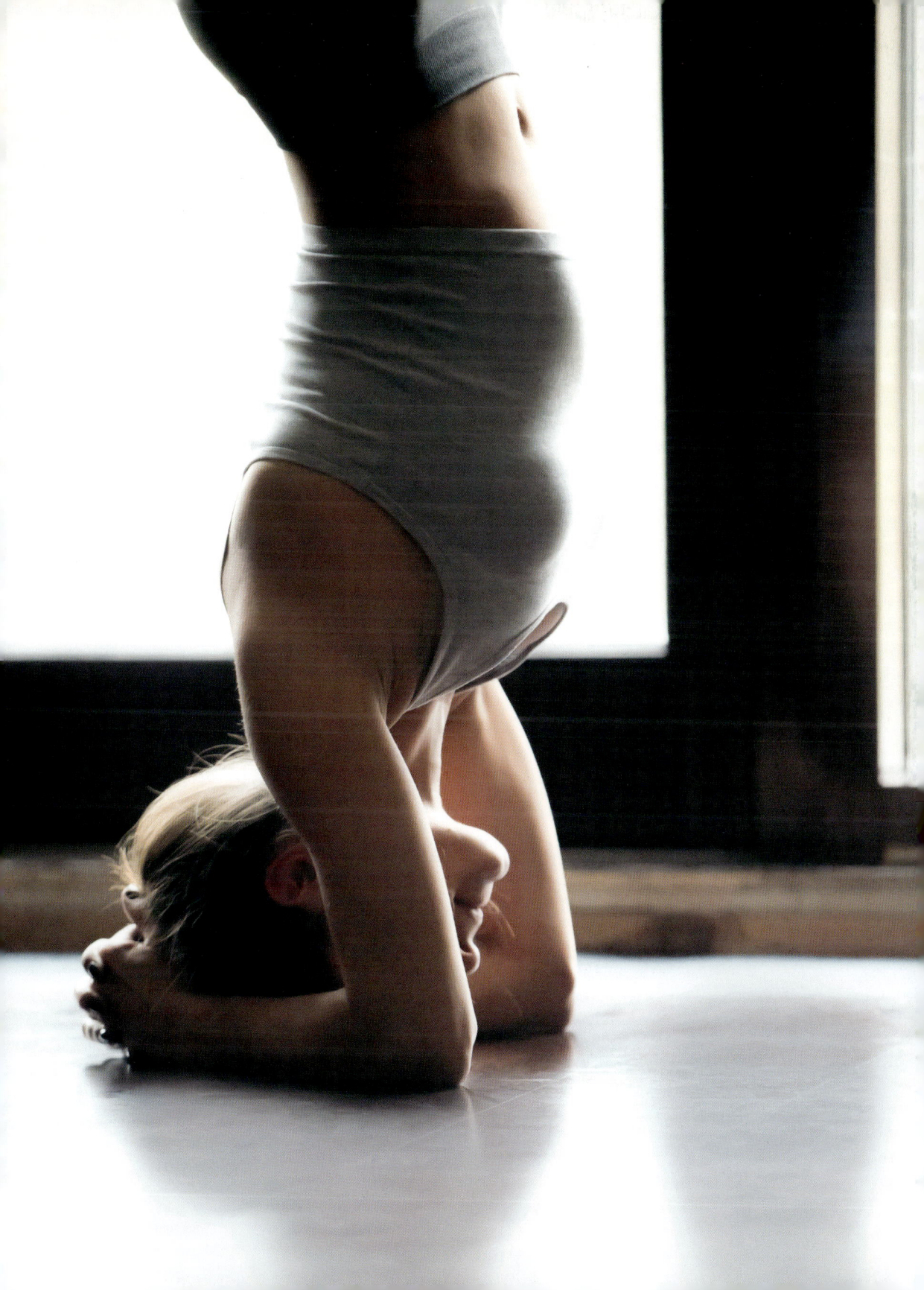

Sirsasana is known as the 'king of postures'. It increases the flow of blood to the brain, rejuvenating its cells and improving their function. The posture also relieves headaches, colds and asthma, and ensures a healthy blood supply to the pituitary and pineal glands, creating a greater sense of well-being and vitality. The inversion of the body helps tired legs and varicose veins, as well as prolapses of the bladder and uterus.

Caution: Don't attempt headstand postures if you have high blood pressure, neck problems, heart problems, thrombosis, chronic catarrh, chronic constipation, detached retina or glaucoma – or if you're overweight.

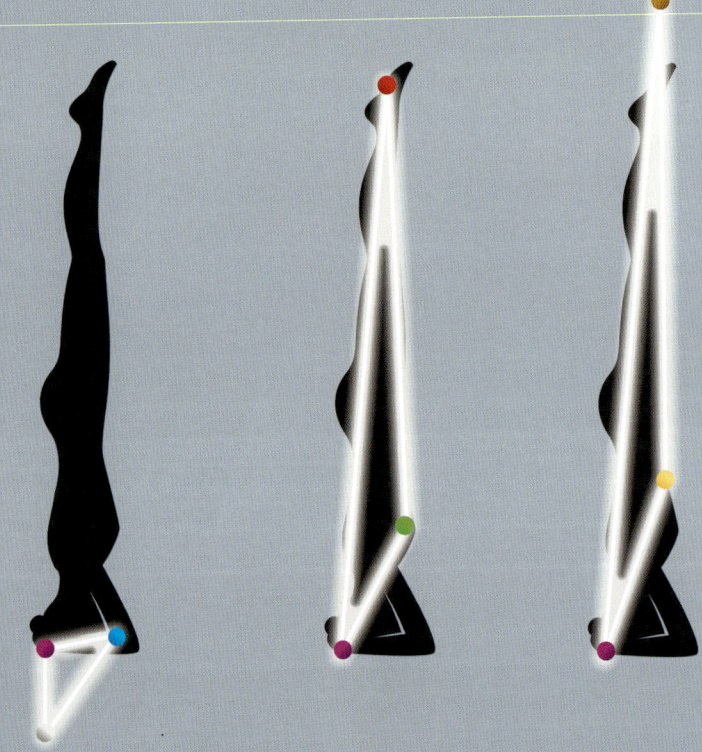

In the full posture (see opposite), three triangles are formed. The first – present on both sides of the body – is with the soul star chakra, the crown chakra and the minor chakra in the crease of the elbow. The second triangle – also present on both sides of the body – is made with the heart chakra, the minor chakra on the sole of the foot and the crown chakra. The third triangle is created with the crown chakra, the earth chakra and the solar plexus chakra.

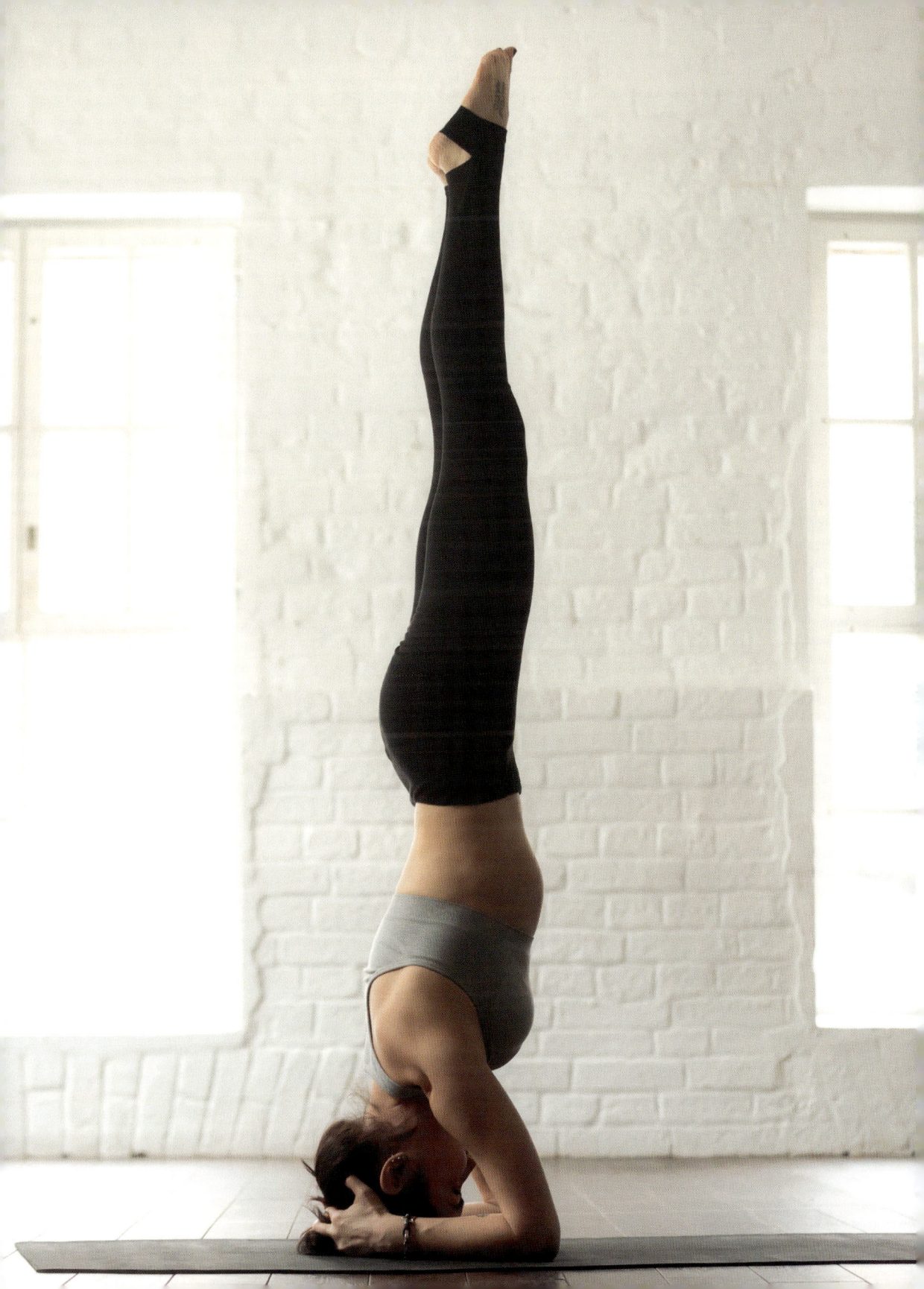

SALAMBA SIRSASANA
(supported headstand)

Practise this headstand against a wall until you've mastered its balance. Kneel on the floor and follow the instructions for bakasana, the crane posture (see page 146). From bakasana, lift your legs up straight until you come into the head balance (see opposite). Hold the posture for approximately 30 seconds to start with, gradually increasing the time until you can hold for 20 minutes. When you're ready, exhale and bring your legs back to bakasana, then back to the kneeling posture. Relax in child's pose (see page 148) for a few minutes.

Salamba sirsasana has the same benefits and cautions as sirsasana (see page 148). The supported headstand also has the additional benefit of strengthening the abdominal muscles through the raising and lowering of the legs into and out of bakasana. Both headstand postures work with the crown chakra.

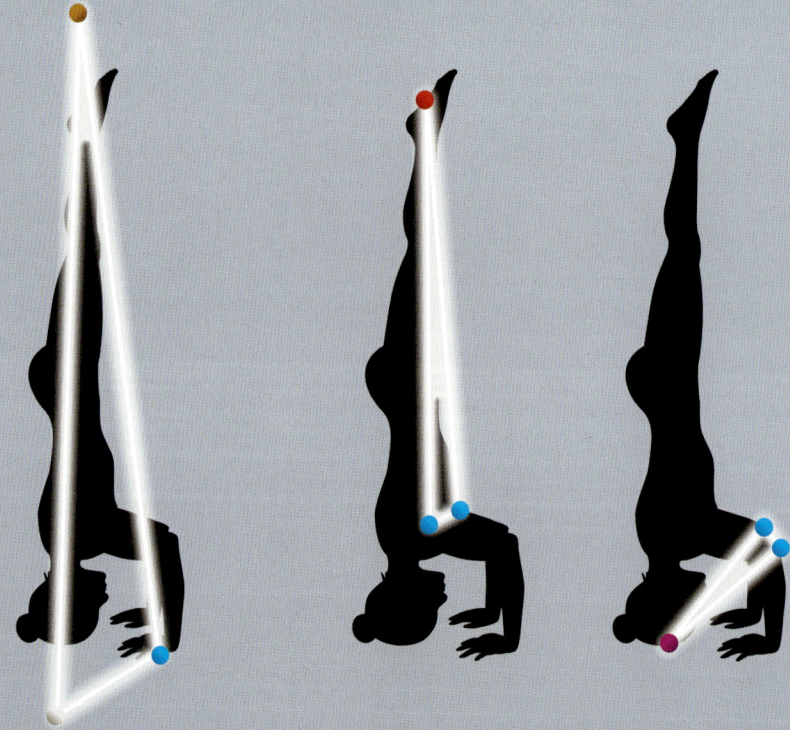

Three main triangles of light are formed in this posture. The first – present on both sides of the body – is with the soul star chakra, the earth chakra and the minor chakra on the palm of the hand. The second triangle – also present on both sides of the body – is made with the minor chakra on the sole of the foot and the minor chakra halfway along each clavicle bone. The third triangle is created with the crown chakra and the minor chakra in the crease of each elbow.

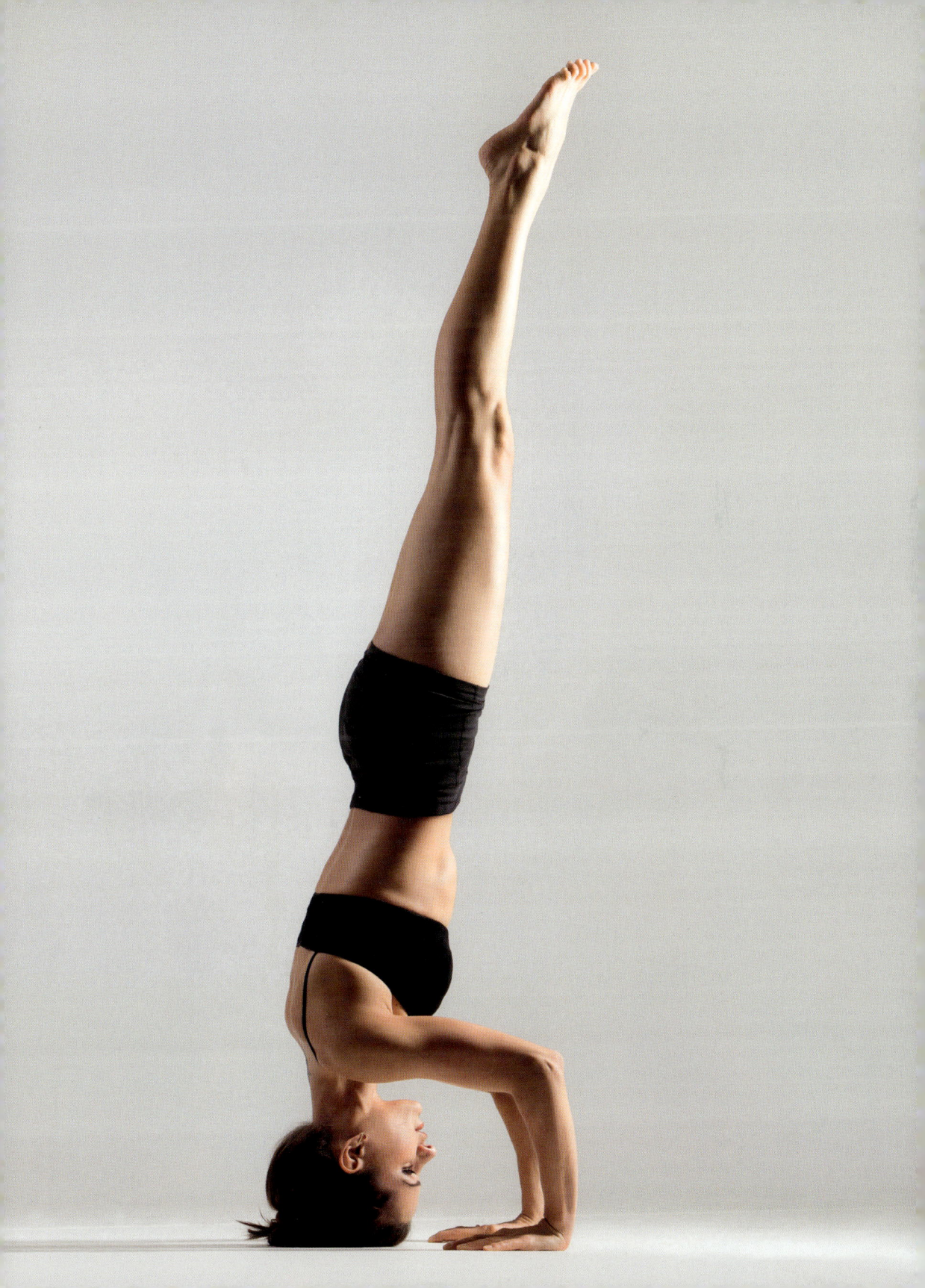

HALASANA (plough posture)

Lie flat on the floor, with your arms by the side of your body, palms facing downwards. Make sure that your neck is extended, with your chin tucked in towards your chest in the chin lock position (see page 80). On the next inhalation, raise your legs – keeping them straight – to 90 degrees. If you find this difficult, bend your knees and then raise your legs. Inhale, and on the next exhalation take your legs over your head until your feet touch the floor behind your head. Lift up your spine until it's straight and then take your hands behind your back and clasp them (see opposite). Hold the posture for as long as is comfortable.

If you can't touch the floor with your feet, place either a folded blanket or books under your feet. If your back is stiff, position a chair behind your head and place your feet on the chair. If you've had an injury to your cervical spine – whiplash, for example – or you suffer a stiff neck, then place folded blankets under your shoulders, resting your head on the floor. This doesn't allow for the chin lock but takes pressure off the cervical spine. .

The plough helps to make the spine and back muscles supple, which benefits the spinal nerves. It also regulates the thyroid gland and balances the metabolic rate, tones the organs of the abdomen – especially the kidneys, liver and pancreas – relieves constipation and removes fat from the waist. The main chakra worked with is the throat chakra – provided you can put on the chin lock.

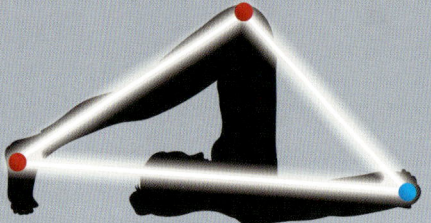

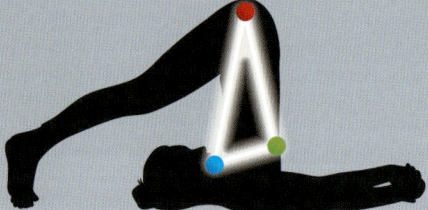

Three main triangles of light are formed in this posture. The first (above), present on both sides of the body, is made with the base chakra, the minor chakra on the sole of the foot and the minor chakra on the palm of each hand. The second triangle (above right) is made with the heart chakra, the base chakra and the throat chakra. The third triangle (right) is created with the solar plexus chakra, the soul star chakra and the throat chakra.

If you have a stiff or injured neck, use blankets when you practise the posture. Fold the blankets and place them on top of each other until you reach the best height. Place your shoulders and back on the blankets, allowing the head and neck to be clear of the blankets and rest on the floor. Now go into the posture. This action allows the neck to be free, and so eliminates any strain.

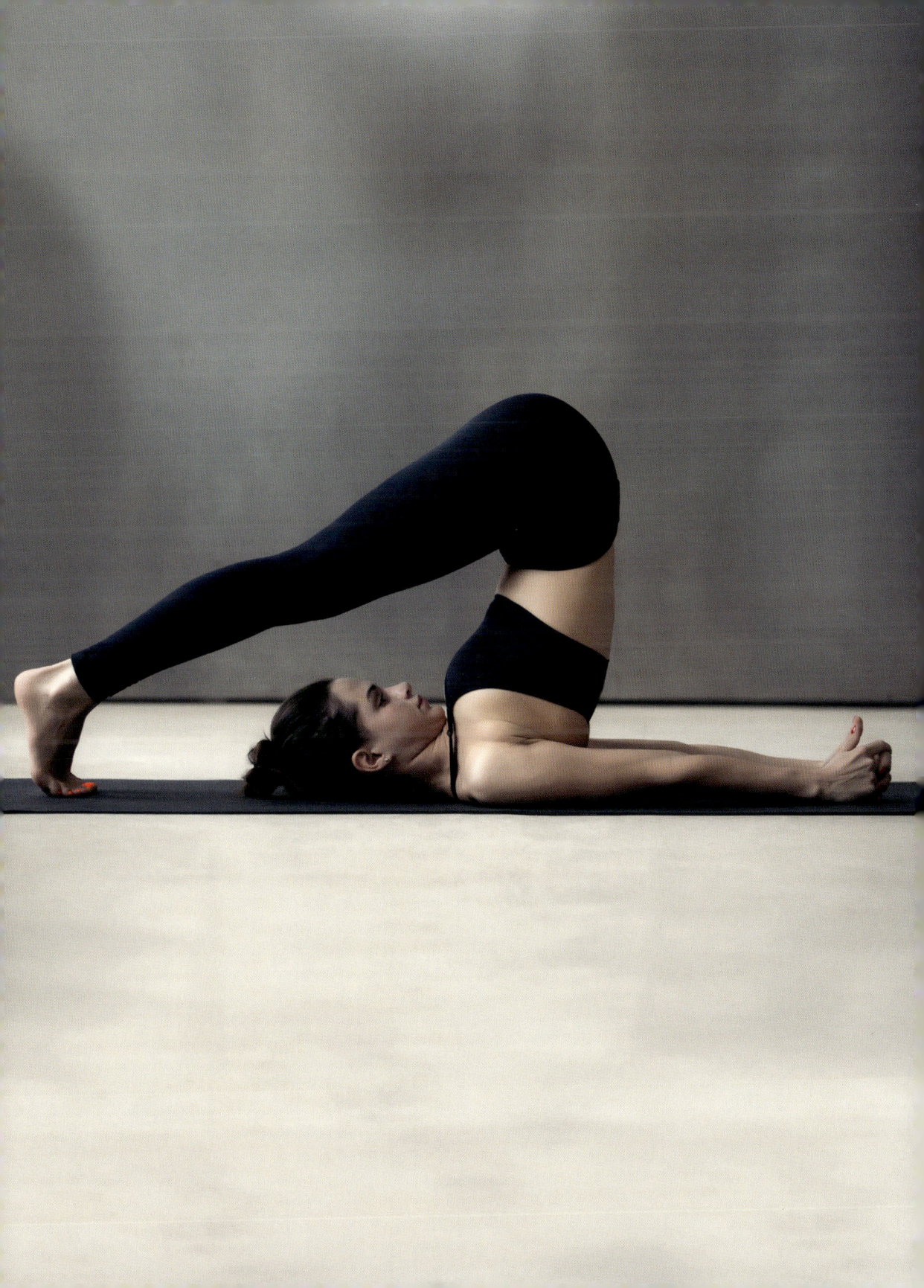

SARVANGASANA (shoulder stand)

Go into halasana (see page 154), then, on an inhalation, raise your legs above your head until your body is in a straight line, from shoulders to toes. With your arms parallel and in line with your shoulders, support your back with your hands (see opposite). It's important that your neck is extended and your chin tucked into your chest to form the chin lock (see page 80). Ensure there's no strain on the cervical spine. If your spine or back are stiff, or you've had an injury to your cervical spine, use blankets as described for halasana. In this posture, you're aiming to straighten the spine – balancing on your shoulders, not on your dorsal spine.

Sarvangasana is often known as the 'mother of postures', because it brings harmony into the physical body. The chin lock in the shoulder balance increases the blood supply to the thyroid gland, thereby helping to regulate its secretions. These secretions have a direct bearing on the reproductive system and also on the hormonal secretions from some of the other endocrine glands. Also, due to the inversion of the body, more blood circulates around the head and chest, which helps those who suffer from bronchitis, asthma or throat problems. With regular practice, you'll feel greater vitality in your body. The chakra that the shoulder stand works with is the throat chakra.

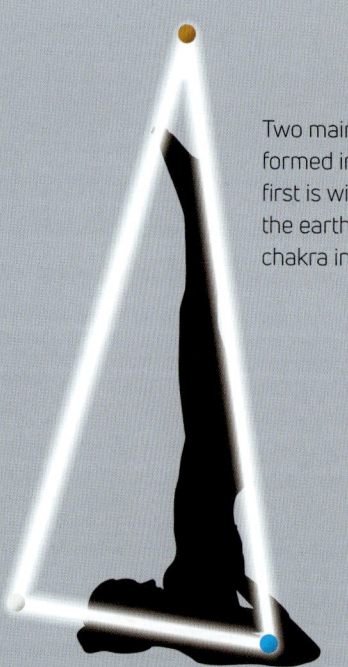

Two main triangles of light are formed in shoulder stand. The first is with the soul star chakra, the earth chakra and the minor chakra in the crease of the elbow.

The second triangle is formed with the minor chakra on the sole of the foot, the throat chakra and the minor chakra in the crease of the arm. These triangles of light are formed on both sides of the body.

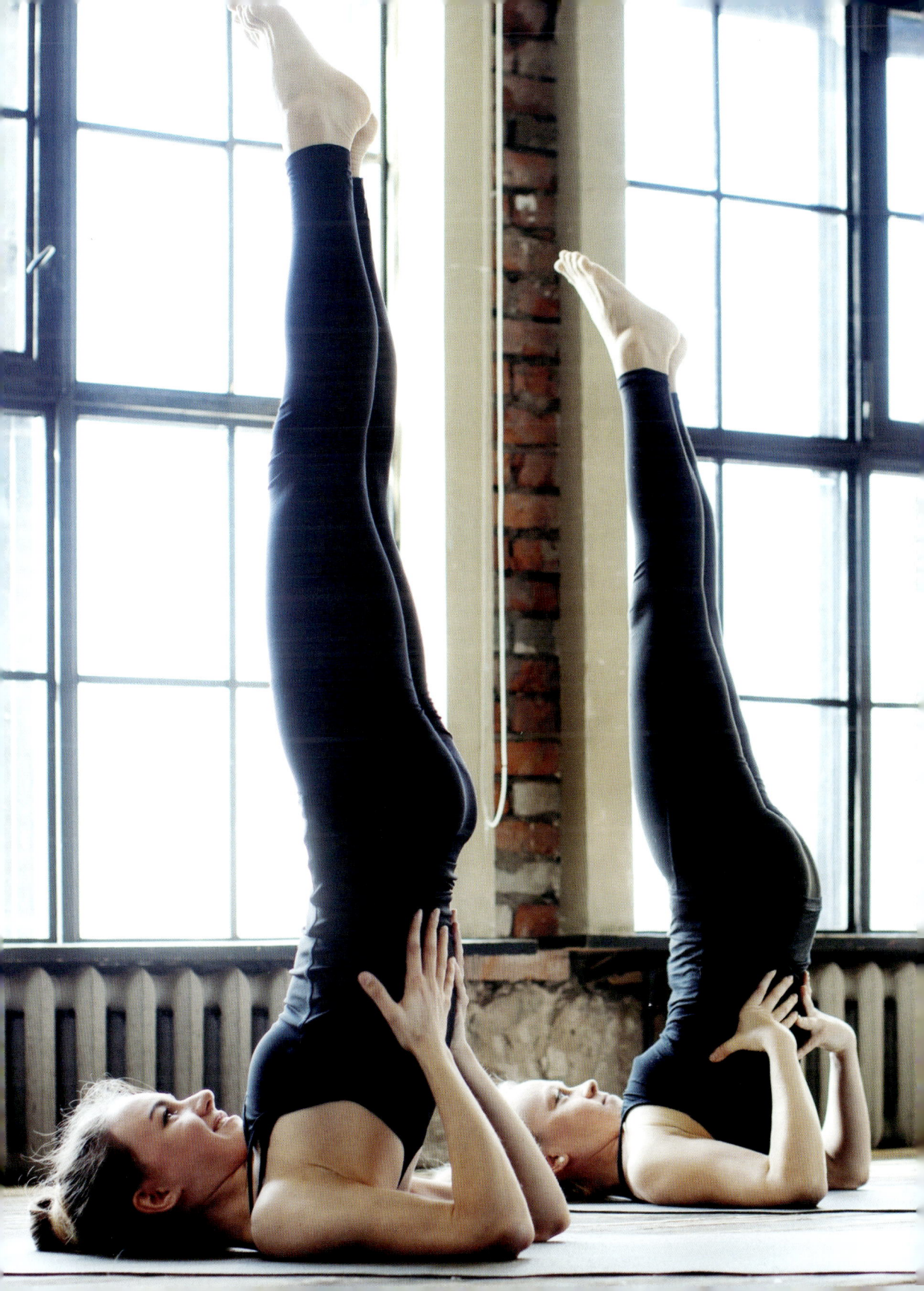

Index

abdominal breathing 58–59
acupuncture points 32, 33
adho mukha svanasana
(dog posture) 112–113
ahimsa (non-violence) 12,
20, 26, 70
Aïvanhov, Omraam Mikhaël
13
ajna see brow chakra
akashic records 24
alta major chakra 6, 38, 52,
80–81
posture 80–81
alternate-nostril breathing
60
anahata see heart chakra
anahata asana (heart
posture) 106–107
angle posture 98–99
apana (downward-flowing
vitality) 43
aparigraha (non-
acquisitiveness) 13
ardha chandrasana (half-
moon posture) 130–131
ardha matsyendrasana (half
spinal twist) 102–103
asanas (postures) 6, 16, 20
holding the posture 20, 32
physical and mental
benefits 16
practising 20
preparation for 20, 32
working with the
triangles of light 90
see also backbends;
inverted postures;
sitting postures;
standing postures
asteya (non-stealing) 12
astral body 35
astral travel 49
attentiveness to God (isvara
pranidhana) 15
aum 46, 48
aura 28, 33–37, 51
layers 33, 35, 37
austerity and spiritual
practice (tapas) 14

backbends
bhujangasana asana
(cobra posture) 138–139
dhanurasana (bow
posture) 140–141

salabhasana (locust
posture) 134–135
supta virasana (reclined
hero posture) 132–133
urdhva dhanurasana
(wheel posture) 144–145
utrasana (camel posture)
136–137
uttana mayurasana
(bridge posture) 142–143
bakasana (crane posture)
146–147
base chakra 13, 33, 41, 46
posture 72–73
visualization 73
Bhagavad-Gita 10, 20
bhujangasana asana (cobra
posture) 138–139
bliss, state of 16, 19, 83
boat posture 104–105
bow posture 140–141
Braden, Gregg 24
bramacharya (chastity) 12–13
breathing
breath control see
pranayama
deep 58
hyperventilation 58
shallow 58
breathing exercises 54–67
abdominal breathing
58–59
alternate-nostril
breathing 60
chest breathing 59
cooling breath 62
humming breath 62
viloma pranayama 64
yoga complete breath 59
bridge posture 142–143
brow chakra 35, 48–49,
51, 52
meditation 83
posture 82
visualization 83
Buddha 35, 56

camel posture 136–137
chakras 16, 30–53, 70
alta major chakra 6, 38,
52, 80–81
base chakra 13, 33, 41, 46,
72–73
brow chakra 35, 48–49,
51, 52, 82–83

chakra clearing 6, 16,
32, 38
crown chakra 48, 50–51,
84–85
earth star chakra 40,
86–87
heart chakra 44–45, 46,
78–79, 90
major chakras 32, 33,
38–52
minor chakras 32, 33, 53,
91
sacral chakra 42, 46, 74–75
solar plexus chakra 43,
46, 76–77
soul star chakra 52,
86–87, 91
throat chakra 46–47, 80–81
chastity (bramacharya) 12–13
chest breathing 59
chitrini nadi 35
the Christ 19, 28, 37, 48, 56
cleanliness (saucha) 14
clothing 58, 70
cobra posture 138–139
concentration (dharana) 18
consciousness, higher 10, 16,
19, 46, 50, 82
contentment (santosa) 14
control of the senses
(pratyahara) 18
cooling breath 62
crane posture 146–147
crown chakra 48, 50–51
posture 84–85
visualization 84

dhanurasana (bow posture)
140–141
dharana (concentration) 18
dhyana (meditation) 6, 10,
15, 19, 57
diet 14
Divine Matrix 24
DNA 24, 28, 40
dodecahedron 28
dog posture 112–113

earth star chakra 40
posture 86–87
Einstein, Albert 24
electromagnetic field see
aura
endocrine system 38, 41, 43,
45, 49

energizing relaxation
technique 91
energy lines 6
see also triangles of light
ether 24, 28, 46
etheric double 33
ethical disciplines (yamas)
12–13
expanded foot posture 118
extended hand to toe
posture 110–111

fifth dimension 90
Francis of Assisi, St 26

Gopi Krishna 50

halasana (plough posture)
154–155
half spinal twist 102–103
half-moon posture 130–131
hand to foot posture
126–127
hanumanasana (the splits)
108–109
head to knee posture
96–97
headstand 148–151
supported headstand
152–153
heart chakra 44–45, 46, 90
posture 78
visualization 78–79
heart posture 106–107
hormonal system 32, 38
humming breath 62

ida nadi 33, 35, 48, 57
incarnation 37
intuition 37
inverted postures
bakasana (crane posture)
146–147
halasana (plough
posture) 154–155
salamba sirsasana
(supported headstand)
152–153
sarvangasana (shoulder
stand) 156–157
sirsasana (headstand)
148–151
isvara pranidhana
(attentiveness to God) 15
Iyengar, B.K.S. 14

janu sirsasana (head to knee posture) 96–97
jnana yoga 10

karma 37, 40
Krishnamurti, Jiddu 15
kundalini 13, 35, 41, 50, 57

lam 41
life force (prana) 6, 16, 28, 33, 43, 56
Lipton, Bruce 28
living in the present 16
locust posture 134–135
Lord Shiva's posture 128–129

Maharishi Mahesh Yogi 56
mandalas 19, 50
manipura *see* solar plexus chakra
mantras 19, 48
    aum 46, 48
    lam 41
meditation (dhyana) 6, 10, 15, 19, 57
    brow chakra 83
Mouth of God *see* alta major chakra
muladhara *see* base chakra

nada yoga 46
nadis 28, 32, 33, 35, 43, 48, 57, 58
namaskar (salutation posture) 92–93
nataraja asana (Lord Shiva's posture) 128–129
navasana (boat posture) 104–105
nectar, divine 47
niyamas (rules of conduct) 14–15
non-acquisitiveness (aparigraha) 13
non-stealing (asteya) 12
non-violence (ahimsa) 12, 20, 26, 70

padangusthasana (hand to foot posture) 126–127
parasympathetic nervous system 33
parivrtta trikonasana (revolving triangle posture) 116–117

Patanjali 6, 10, 13
pentagram 28
pingala nadi 33, 35, 48
plough posture 154–155
positive thinking 26, 35
postures (asanas) *see* backbends; inverted postures; sitting postures; standing postures
prana (life force) 6, 16, 28, 33, 43, 56–57
    apana vayu 57
    channelling 56–57
    prana vayu 57
    samana vayu 57
    udana vayu 57
    vyana vayu 57
    white pranic light 62
pranyayama (breath control) 16, 19
    bandhas (body locks) 56–57, 60
    channelling prana 56–57
    exhalation 16
    inhalation 16
    retention 16, 58
    see also breathing exercises
prasarita padottanasana (expanded foot posture) 118
pratyahara (control of the senses) 18
present, living in the 18
psychic union posture 94–95
purvottanasana (upward plank posture) 100–101

reclined hero posture 132–133
reverse virabhadrasana (reverse warrior posture) 124–125
reverse warrior posture 124–125
revolving triangle posture 116–117
Rig Veda 23
rules of conduct (niyamas) 14–15

sacral chakra 42, 46
    posture 74–75
    visualization 75

sacred geometry 28
sahasrara *see* crown chakra
Sai Baba 28
salabhasana (locust posture) 134–135
salamba sirsasana (supported headstand) 152–153
salutation posture 92–93
samadhi (self-realization) 10, 14, 19, 37
santosa (contentment) 14
sarvangasana (shoulder stand) 156–157
satya (truthfulness) 12
saucha (cleanliness) 14
self-realization (samadhi) 10, 14, 19, 37
self-study (svadhyaya) 15
shoulder stand 156–157
sirsasana (headstand) 148–151
sitting postures
    anahata asana (heart posture) 106–107
    ardha matsyendrasana (half spinal twist) 102–103
    hanumanasana (the splits) 108–109
    janu sirsasana (head to knee posture) 96–97
    namaskar (salutation posture) 92–93
    navasana (boat posture) 104–105
    purvottanasana (upward plank posture) 100–101
    upavistha konasana (angle posture) 98–99
    yoga mudrasana (psychic union posture) 94–95
solar plexus chakra 43, 46
    posture 76
    visualization 77
soul star chakra 52, 91
    posture 86–87
sound 46
    primordial sound (anahata sound) 44, 46
splits 108–109
standing postures
    adho mukha svanasana (dog posture) 112–113
    ardha chandrasana (half-moon posture) 130–131

nataraja asana (Lord Shiva's posture) 128–129
padangusthasana (hand to foot posture) 126–127
parivrtta trikonasana (revolving triangle posture) 116–117
prasarita padottanasana (expanded foot posture) 118
reverse virabhadrasana (reverse warrior posture) 124–125
trikonasana (triangle posture) 114–115
utthita hasta padangusthasana (extended hand to toe posture) 110–111
virabhadrasana 1 (warrior posture 1) 120–121
virabhadrasana 2 (warrior posture 2) 122–123
supported headstand 152–153
supta virasana (reclined hero posture) 132–133
sushumna nadi 35, 41, 48, 57
sutras 10
svadhyaya (self-study) 15
svadisthana *see* sacral chakra
swastika 43
sympathetic nervous system 35

tantric yoga 13
tapas (austerity and spiritual practice) 14
telepathy 49
third eye 48
thought, power of 28
    see also positive thinking
throat chakra 46–47
    posture 80–81
Tolle, Ekhart 18
Transcendental Meditation 56
triangle posture 114–115
    revolving triangle posture 116–117

continued overleaf ▶

Index

triangles of light 6, 7, 16, 28, 32, 33, 38, 88–91
  energizing relaxation technique 91
  visualization 32, 90, 91
  working with 90–91
  see also specific asanas (postures)
trikonasana (triangle posture) 114–115
truthfulness (satya) 12

Upanishads 10
upavistha konasana (angle posture) 98–99
upward plank posture 100–101
urdhva dhanurasana (wheel posture) 144–145
utrasana (camel posture) 136–137

uttana mayurasana (bridge posture) 142–143
utthita hasta padangusthasana (extended hand to toe posture) 110–111

vajra nadi 35
viloma pranayama (breathing exercise) 64
virabhadrasana 1 (warrior posture 1) 120–121
virabhadrasana 2 (warrior posture 2) 122–123
visshudha *see* throat chakra
visualization 19, 32
  base chakra 73
  brow chakra 83
  crown chakra 84
  heart chakra 78–79

sacral chakra 75
solar plexus chakra 77
soul star and earth chakras 86
triangles of light 32, 90, 91
white pranic light 62

Walsh, Neale Donald 37
warming up 32, 70, 71–80
warrior
  reverse warrior posture 124–125
  warrior posture 1 120–121
  warrior posture 2 122–123
web of light 24–28, 33
  accessing 24
  in action 24, 26
wheel of life 50
wheel posture 144–145

yamas (ethical disciplines) 12–13
yoga
  eight yogic steps 6, 10, 12–19, 20
  jnana yoga 10
  story and essence of 10
yoga complete breath 59
yoga mudrasana (psychic union posture) 94–95
yoga practice
  accessories 70
  clothing 70
  food and water 70
  location 70
  routine 70
  warming up 32, 70
  see also asanas (postures)
Yoga Sutras 10
Yogananda, Paramahansa 12, 15, 18

PICTURE CREDITS

Cover fizkes/ShutterStockphoto.Inc; author photograph Bipin Dattani

ShutterStockphoto.Inc 2 -3 F8 studio; 7 Kite_rin; 8 Rovenko Photo; 11, 12 Kudryashka; 13 Rawpixel.com; 14 Kudryashka; 15 Rawpixel.com; 16 Kudryashka; 17 fizkes; 18 Kudryashka; 19 Rawpixel.com; 20 Kudryashka; 21 Rawpixel.com; 25 sumkinn; 27 norph; 34 Jacky Brown; 36 Titima Ongkantong; 39 Reamolko; 54-5 exile_artist; 61, 63, 65, 66-7 fizkes; 68-9 codesyn; 73, 74, 76, 82, 85, 87 fizkes; 88-9 F8 studio; 94 fizkes; 97 Evgeny Glazunov; 98, 101, 103 fizkes; 107 LightField Studios; 109 fizkes; 111 Evgeny Glazunov; 113, 115, 117, 121, 123, 125, 127, 129, 133, 135, 137 fizkes; 139 bezikus; 141, 143 Evgeny Glazunov; 145 fizkes; 147 Viktor Gladkov; 149, 151, 153, 155 fizkes;

iStockphoto 105 yulkapopkova

Getty Images 93, 119, 131, 157 PeopleImages

Foliage image Reece with a C/ShutterStockphoto.Inc
Silhouettes images ShutterStockphoto.Inc; Fogdog

ACKNOWLEDGEMENTS

Eddison Books Limited
Managing Director Lisa Dyer
Managing Editor Tessa Monina
Designed and edited by Fogdog Creative (www.fogdog.co.uk)
Proofreader Jane Roe
Indexer Marie Lorimer
Production Sarah Rooney & Cara Clapham